I0421117

Paleo Diet

How you can eat a Paleo Diet on a Budget without Going Broke

(25 Slow Cook Recipes and Desserts)

By Malik Johnson

Table of Contents

INTRODUCTION:
Paleo Diet: Introduction to a Way of Life that's as old as Humanity Itself

The Hunter Vs The Hunted: Which One Do You Want to Be?

I'd like to introduce you to two different types-ancient man and modern man. Ancient man (and woman!) was a strong, healthy, alert hunter who was on top of the food chain. Modern man has lost the natural survival instincts and skills to be the sharp, fit and vigorous hunters that our ancient ancestors were. Instead modern man has become the hunted, a weak, sick, overweight and exhausted prey that is no longer a survivor. Let's take a look at how the hunted modern man compares to the ancient hunter.

Modern man has a hard time waking up in the morning. He has to hit the snooze button a couple of times before he can finally manage to drag himself out of bed. He stands up unsteadily, feeling aches and pains in his joints, bones and muscles as he staggers into the bathroom. Once there, he might catch a glimpse of his reflection in the bathroom mirror and be unpleasantly surprised by what he sees: An exhausted expression, bleary eyes ringed with dark, unhealthy looking under eye circles, dull, lifeless looking skin and prematurely graying or receding hair and a bloated body that just keeps piling on the pounds no matter how hard he tries to eat healthy. If that's the reflection that also faced you in the mirror this morning, then you are like millions of other Americans who seem to be growing sick, fat, tired and older than their age, at breakneck speed. But what's behind this epidemic of illness and weight gain, you may be wondering. Let's take a look at the next step of modern man's morning routine for clues as to the most likely culprit.

At some point during the morning rush, modern man stops for a quick breakfast and grabs whatever is convenient. This usually means packaged, highly processed breakfast foods like frozen waffles, pop tarts or other "hearty" breakfast pastry goods with enough sugar in them to make him feel momentarily awake and energized. Then again, perhaps he will choose something more health conscious and opt for a better, more nutritionally balanced meal, like the kind promoted by the food pyramid: something like a bowl of "healthy" whole wheat cereal and some low-fat milk, a granola bar or a multi-grain bagel (without any butter), all washed down with a nice, tall glass of orange, or some other packaged fruit juice.

Modern man is often concerned about health and listens to the advice of conventional nutritionists and doctors, so he probably feels that he's done a great job choosing the second type of breakfast. In fact, as long as he steers clear of so-called dangerous foods like eggs, butter, fatty meats and keeps everything in his fridge, from yogurt to milk, strictly low-fat or fat-free, nutritionists, doctors and dieticians will tell him that he's eating a healthy diet and has nothing to worry about.

So if that's true, why does he feel so tired, even after that "energizing" breakfast? Why is it difficult for him to even climb into his car and drive to the office and why does he feel like he's run a marathon by the time he sits down at his desk? He's not alone there, either. This is why coffee has become the nation's number one fuel, helping people to get through hours of seated work. During his long workday, the few times he'll get up, other than bathroom breaks, will be in order to re-fill his mug of sugary coffee or stock up on some quick, high-calorie, processed snacks, because his "super-nutritious" breakfast and heavy lunch have actually left him feeling completely exhausted and wiped out.

By the time modern man's workday is over, he is thoroughly drained of all energy and can only drive home and collapse on the couch with a rushed fast-food dinner. He will probably stay on the computer or watch television late into the night and when he does finally climb into bed, he will most likely find it hard to get to sleep. The next morning, the poor quality of his sleep will catch up with him as he struggles to find the strength to roll out of bed all over again.

When it comes to health, modern man suffers all kinds of non-communicable diseases and conditions that ancient man has never heard of. Modern man is a victim of everything from diabetes to autoimmune disorders, different types of cancer and cardiovascular diseases to organ failure and dementia and is constantly being hunted by the rising risk of obesity, premature aging and depression. He spends a huge portion of his income on medical care and expensive prescription drugs but he only gets sicker, more tired, more overweight and unhealthier with every dollar he spends. Does this sound familiar?

If it does, that's because the routine I just described is extremely common nowadays. In fact, being weak, exhausted, ill and overweight has become the norm, not the exception for most people. But it wasn't always this way. Once, the average human was a lean, well-muscled, quick-thinking, agile and well-balanced survivor- at the top of the game and the food chain mentally, physically and emotionally. This kind of ancient human, let's call him the Hunter,(or the huntress, as the case may be) lived a totally different life than we do today and it is this lifestyle that is the secret to the Hunter's health, vigor and fitness. Let's take a look at how the Hunter's daily routine compares to the modern man's routine:

The Hunter was an early riser. As the sun came up, the Hunter would instinctively rise as well, because his body was still in tune with the natural rhythms of nature. He would spring up easily from the ground where he slept without having to struggle or fight off drowsiness. Because his health was at optimal levels, he was able to wake up alert, energetic and prepared to protect himself from any threats in his environment. The Hunter's morning routine did not include a large, carbohydrate-filled breakfast like ours often do today. Instead, he would have eaten(if he was hungry) a light, animal protein rich meal such as a handful of leftovers from the previous evening's dinner, drank from his store of clean, pure water and headed out into the wild, for a full day of outdoor activity. As a hunter, he would have relied on his health, fitness and alertness every day to ensure his own survival and that of his family unit, meaning that he was typically responsible for bringing home vital food supplies.

Unlike the modern man who is a prisoner to an inactive desk job, the Hunter would therefore spend a large portion of his day stalking and hunting in the sun and fresh air. This would only increase his health and energy as he absorbed vital vitamin D from the sun's rays and got plenty of natural intermittent exercise from his stop-and-start movements. The Hunter was not tied to ridiculous and unnatural food rules like the ones we are taught by nutritionists and conventional doctors these days so he would eat sparingly throughout the day, neither over-snacking nor worrying about stuffing down large meals at precise times. Instead, he would listen to his own body for the cues that would tell him how much food he needed at any given time. The fatty, protein laden morning meal he had eaten earlier would help to nourish his brain and body, giving him a stable source of energy and the mental clarity needed to keep an eye on the animals he was seeking to hunt as well as avoiding threats and dangers like large carnivores, poisonous snakes and insects and dangerous terrain. Because the Hunter was not slowed down by excess weight or flagging energy like the modern man is today, he was able to survive and excel, no matter how challenging his environment was.

By the time the hunting day was done and he had captured his prey, he would still have all the energy required to drag his prize back home to the cooking fire. Unlike modern man, the Hunter lived in perfect harmony with the natural cycle of the day so once it was dark and he had eaten his meal of rich nourishing animal proteins and fats along with perhaps a handful of seeds or wild grown vegetables, he would begin to slip into a meditative, calm state, ready for a deeply revitalizing, healing sleep. As he slept, the Hunter didn't have to worry about being woken by a beeping cell phone or flashing lights from electronic gadgets like we do today. He was able to rest in total darkness, allowing his body to repair and restore every tissue and cell to perfect working order, preventing damage and disease and helping him to wake, ready to face any challenges the next day.

Modern man faces many challenges today, but most of them are within his power to change while our ancestor the Hunter was surrounded by many unpredictable challenges and dangers. Still, modern man is failing miserably at meeting his challenges while the Hunter successfully beat all of the odds and not only survived but

THRIVED in his difficult environment. Modern man is a victim while ancient man was a victor. Modern man is HUNTED by illness, obesity, exhaustion and depression while ancient man was the ultimate HUNTER. Why? The answer is quite simply the Paleolithic lifestyle. Living in a Paleolithic (Paleo for short) way means the difference between being lean , healthy and active and being tired, ill and overweight,. It's the difference between having wonderful mental clarity and alertness or always feeling like your thinking is somehow cloudy and slow. Paleo is not just about weight loss. Yes, you will definitely lose any excess weight and easily attain the most balanced and physically fit body possible with this lifestyle but it provides benefits that go far beyond just that. In fact, Paleo living can do everything from improve your health, prevent diseases like type 2 diabetes, autoimmune disorders, cardiovascular and neurological diseases to heal and treat systemic candida infections, give your sharper thinking and reactions and even clear your skin.

Paleo is NOT a diet. It is a lifestyle shift that unleashes the inner hunter in you, providing you with the ability to naturally become the best, quickest, fittest, strongest and healthiest versions of ourselves that you can be. Paleo is NOT another fad-diet that pushes you to purchase a lot of expensive, low- nutrient, high-carb, sugary and chemical laden packaged "diet" foods. It is an amazingly powerful way of eating, drinking, exercising and being that WORKS because it is basically a step-by-step return to the healthy, fit and strong state humans used to exist in-and best of all, it doesn't have to be expensive. If you are looking for a way to completely transform your body, mind and energy levels but you're worried about investing in a lot of costly diet items and exercise gear, then Paleo is definitely for you! Paleo is all about using what's at hand to sharpen and hone your body and mind until you are at the peak of physical and mental fitness, just as our hunter-gatherers used what was available to them to become the ultimate survivors. If you've had enough of all of the conventional and misleading nutrition and fitness advice that has made modern humans so out of shape, overweight, exhausted and sick, if you're ready to bypass the expensive gimmicky diets that NEVER really work, if you want to see yourself transformed into the most elite, most skilled, strong, fit and healthy you possible-WITHOUT wasting time or money, then you are definitely ready for PALEO.

Let's get started!

Chapter 1:
What is Paleo?

The Paleo (Paleolithic) diet, also known as the caveman diet, is a way of eating that tries to match the ancestral eating habits of the human race as closely as possible, in order to improve health and maximize fitness. The paleo diet is based on the fact that while we may have learned many things since the end of our ancient hunting and gathering societies, proper nutrition is not one of them. While modern day humans are more sophisticated and technologically advanced (and better groomed!), our ancient ancestors definitely beat us in the health, nutrition and fitness categories. Our modern day diets are stuffed with harmful ingredients and our health, weight and brains are suffering under the strain of the "modern" diseases like obesity, cardiovascular diseases, high blood pressure, diabetes, autoimmune disorders and dementia. The Paleo diet's main foundation is built on foods that our ancient hunter-gatherer ancestors would have eaten, such as meats, eggs, fats, nuts, seeds, greens and berries while it excludes the often dangerous and unnecessary foods that our ancestors never ate but form a big part of our poor diets today, such as grains of all kinds, refined sugars, processed foods with unnatural chemicals, additives and industrial cooking oils. Because ancient humans never had access to such items and because, despite the time gap between them and us, modern humans' bodies are still made the same way, it stands to reason that the foods our ancestors never ate is food we shouldn't be eating either. On the other hand, the foods that cavemen ate in abundance are nourishing, energy and life-sustaining foods that we no longer eat in the quantities we should. And what are the results?

With every passing generation, the human body is becoming weaker, more broken down, less-muscled, less-balanced, more overweight and diseases-riddled. The human brain is being attacked on all sides by artificial stimulation, stress, chemicals and sugars, resulting in cloudy thinking, memory loss and even complete loss of cognitive abilities.

While our ancient ancestors could hunt large animals with only a spear, we are too weak to climb up a flight of stairs. While our ancient ancestors could comfortably walk many miles through rough terrain, bare foot, we can't even imagine going 2 blocks down the road without a car. Ancient hunter-gatherers could calculate the dangers in a situation at lightning speed, making quick, life-saving decisions at the drop of a pin but today, we are losing the gift of speedy thinking and have a hard time remembering even familiar names and numbers.

While our ancient ancestors ate to the full, deeply enjoying their protein and nutrient rich real food while staying slim, ultra-fit and healthy, we are constantly counting calories, feeling guilty about every bite we eat, trying diet after diet and still piling on stubborn pounds, no matter what we do! Which one sounds like a healthy, beneficial diet to you? In fact, if you dropped those ancient hunters into our modern environment today, they might struggle to get used to the fast-paced, high-stress way we live and have some difficulty getting understanding our technology but on the whole, with their well-nourished, fast-thinking minds and healthy, agile, disease-resistant bodies, they would adapt much better than the average overweight, under-nourished, ill and out of shape modern human would if dropped into the wilderness.

So at its root, Paleo is basically about making a choice between survival and extinction, thriving and failing, fitness, health and strength or flabbiness, illness and weakness. It's about turning the clock back on your fatigued, ailing and weight-saddled body and going from being the victim of modern foods, diseases and stress to being the victor.

The choice is yours. Which one do you want to be-the hunter or the hunted? If you choose to be the hunter, then rest assured that you've come to the right place. The Paleo way of eating was voted the most effective diet of all time by thousands of people who've tied it worldwide for a very good reason-it REALLY works. Not in a "lose 5 pounds, put 2 back on, kind-of-feel-better" sort of way. No, when I say it works, I mean it works in a "completely change your body, lose and keep off all excess weight, get fitter, faster, stronger, leaner, feel better than you've ever felt before" kind of way! If that sounds good to you, then there's nothing left to do but get started:

Paleo improves your well-being, health, body weight and fitness by allowing you to eat REAL foods and cutting out all of the ARTIFICIAL, non-nourishing, damaging food items your body was never meant to consume.

Let's look at what foods should make up the bulk of your Paleo meal plan:

- Vegetables

- Meats

- Fish

- Eggs

- Fruits

- Nuts

- Seeds

And the items that you should strictly avoid on your Paleo eating plan are:

- Sugar

- Grains

- Artificial flavors, colors and additives

- All processed foods and beverages

- Legumes

Because Paleo is not a "diet" in the gimmicky, "eat only one or two types of food for a month" sense, it does allow you a large scope for personal choices and preferences as long as you are truly listening to your body and honoring its reactions and sensitivities. That's why certain foods are left in a sort of "free zone", meaning you can choose whether to add them into your diet at all, eliminate them completely or limit their intake, depending on your own unique reaction and tolerance level:

These foods include:

- Dairy products

- Certain starchy vegetables

So now that we've got the most basic components Paleo down, you may be thinking: Isn't this going to be really expensive? I can tell you right away that you DO NOT need to spend tons of money to eat a successful and effective Paleo meal plan. In fact, many people find that, when they cut out all of the unnecessary spending on harmful, unnatural and super-fattening packaged foods and drinks, they actually end up putting more away in the bank each month than they ever did before they went Paleo. Not to mention all of the money that is saved from unpleasant and unfruitful medical spending as a result of your new diet that eliminates and prevents a huge array of diseases and conditions.

And when it comes to exercise, because the Paleo way of life is about natural movement and not pounding away on some machine for hours, you don't have to worry about needing to splash out on pricey gym memberships and fancy workout gear to lose weight. And that's why Paleo is such a popular lifestyle and what this book is really about: harnessing all of the benefits of weight loss, health, renewed energy, rejuvenated mind, body and appearance while at the same time finding and using awesome techniques that will save you money and time and generally make this the best, easiest and most natural change you've ever made.

Taking care of your health getting the body you deserve and protecting your mind and physique from the ravages of aging should never be a choice between money and well-being, and with Paleo it's not! Instead, utilize the step-by-step, easy to use advice and information in this book to achieve the health and fitness you desire without wasting a single cent!

Chapter 2:
Great Health Doesn't Have to Break the Bank: Affordable Ways to Go Paleo

The Paleo way of eating is quickly catching on like wildfire, because it provides undeniable results. But the one thing that stands between even more people joining this health movement and gaining the bodies, brains and lives they've always wanted is price.

Many people insist that eating Paleo *has* to be expensive. In fact, it's one of the biggest excuses a lot of people use to justify their unhealthy, carb and sugar-loaded, fast food lifestyle.

That's why I wrote this book. Because the truth is, there is absolutely NO reason why eating Paleo has to cost more than eating the Standard American Diet (SAD). Thousands of people have been shocked by the fact that they are actually SAVING money by eating Paleo. You may be shaking your head in disbelief right now but I promise you that once you've read this guide on eating Paleo on a budget, you will never believe that Paleo is too expensive again. Are you ready to learn the secrets of shedding those pounds and kicking illness and fatigue to the curb for good, without wasting any of your hard-earned cash? If so, read on. I promise, it'll be well-worth your time:

1. **Cut Out The Middle**: What do I mean by this? The next time you go into your local grocery store, take a moment to notice how the items are laid out. You will quickly realize that all of the real food such as the fruits, vegetables, meat and deli counter and the dairy areas are all lining the edge of the grocery store while the conventional, commercially prepared, highly processed junk "food" is given pride of place, right smack dab in the center of the store. In fact, this is why so many people struggle to shop smart and bring home healthy items. These fattening and disease causing products are constantly calling to shoppers from their privileged position in the middle of the store, beckoning you to come and spend your precious dollars on a bunch of chemically enhanced, toxic boxes and bags that will only leave you fat, sick, tired and miserable. So what is the number one rule of Paleo supermarket shopping? CUT OUT THE MIDDLE! That's right, ignore all of those aisles upon aisles of strategically positioned poisons and head

straight for the out perimeter. Make a beeline for the fresh produce section where you can load up on a lot of fresh vegetables and some fruits, then go and stock up on some protein in the meat and deli sections. If you are dairy tolerant, make sure you stop off and pick up some whole fat, grass-fed milk and butter as well as cartons of eggs and then go right to the checkout counter without giving those middle aisles a second glance. I guarantee you that when you hear how little your whole grocery cart of food costs, your jaw will hit the floor. Why? Simply because cutting out the entire middle of the supermarket and ONLY buying real foods means BIG savings. Think about it: How much do you think the average American spends on unhealthy junk foods ranging from sugary, carb-loaded cereal boxes to bags and bags of cookies, chips and other snack items, not to mention dessert items like cakes, packs of donuts, cartons of ice cream and what about beverages? Don't forget all of the cans, jugs and bottles of soft drinks, diet drinks, sports and energy drinks as well as supposedly "healthy" processed fruit juices that most people can't go a single day without. Now remove all of these items from your grocery list. It looks pretty short right? This is the main secret behind why insiders often joke that once you go Paleo, your wallet gets heavier while your body gets lighter!

2. **Eat In:** A lot of Paleo eaters do this anyway, even if they aren't necessarily trying to save money. The simple fact is that it's way easier to create simple, flavorful and delicious Paleo dishes at home for yourself and your family than trying to explain to every waiter you meet that no, pasta is not grain-free or quizzing the chef about just how many chemicals went into his special sauce.

In short, you have to be in control of what goes into your body to truly be an effective Paleo eater. Restaurants may seem like a fast option but in the end they are actually just a fast route to weight gain and health problems. Now let's talk about the money:

A moderately priced meal in the average restaurant can cost up to 15 dollars and if you are eating out even once a day, that really adds up. In one month you would be shelling out $450 on eating out alone and $900 on eating out, if there are two of you!

The same People who claim Paleo is too expensive to be done on a budget are the ones who eat out regularly and when you really think about it, wouldn't you rather feed your body and mind ultra-nourishing, fresh and real food while saving money than waste both money and your health by eating chemically-enhanced "dead" restaurant meals at expensive prices? Now, keep in in mind that just because you've gone Paleo, it doesn't necessarily mean that you CAN'T eat out once in a while. It just means that you have to be more careful with your food selections and choose a restaurant that is honest about its ingredients, so you can ensure that your health is well cared for, at the same time as you enjoy your meal. On the flip side, cook at home way more often and you will find that not only will you see your monthly grocery bill drop drastically but so will your weight. It's a simple fact that commercially prepared meals aren't going to be as cleanly and healthily prepared as your own home cooking, so if you really want to give your body a good shot at getting all of the benefits of going Paleo, limit your restaurant trips and start preparing the food your body really craves at home. If you're worried about learning to cook Paleo, don't be. Simply check out the recipe index at the back of this book for easy, delicious and nutritious Paleo meals you can make in no time flat!

3. **Learn the 80/20 Theory:** Many famous proponents of the Paleo way of eating and living have been doing this for years and while they absolutely love the amazing results of their ancestral lifestyles they also understand that thousands of years have passed since we were hunter-gatherers and the modern world is not going to be as Paleo friendly as the ancient one was. Do they let this stop them from getting all of the benefits of Paleo and enjoying themselves and their lives at the same time? No! In fact, that's where the 80/20 school of thought comes in. The 80/20 principle basically states that as long as you are giving the Paleo way of eating and living a real and committed try and you are staying away from the biggest dietary and lifestyle offenders, you don't have to stress unnecessarily about the one or two times

that modern life has made it difficult or impossible to make the most Paleo choice. For example, what do you do if you have to eat in a restaurant and the grass-fed beef option is too expensve? Simple, you just choose another protein and animal fat rich option like non-grass fed steak or chicken, remove any non-Paleo side dishes and sauces and ENJOY your meal!

Paleo is not about trying to go back thousands of years in the past. That would be impossible and some would say, rather unpleasant, no matter how much money you spend. Instead, it is about harnessing the ancient secrets of eating and living that made hunter-gatherers so much healthier than modern man and using that information as a way to get and stay healthy and fit in today's world. 80/20 basically means that if you're sticking fully to Paleo 80% of the time, then you will see amazing results and get all of the benefits, regardless of the 20% where life happens and you can't always make the best Paleo choice. This theory has helped thousands of people get and stay Paleo because it allows for people with different budgets and different schedules to all get what they need out of Paleo. It's not hard and fast rule, so for instance, you may be able to do 90%perfect Paleo and only have to make compromises 10% of the time. In that case, you're doing great and will see results a little faster but those that are 80/20 will also be getting excellent and life-changing results too. That's the great thing about the Paleo way of eating and living. It really is a lifestyle instead of a fad diet. Paleo doesn't tell you that you have to live off of expensive food like asparagus and lobster, it doesn't mean you have to buy fancy vitamins, supplements and weight loss shakes. It quite simply means living as closely to your body's natural, ancestral way of being as possible. And guess what? Whether you are doing 80/20 or 90/10 or 100%, Paleo really works. It delivers jaw-dropping results in a short amount of time and as long as you don't go back to sugary, carb-loaded, processed eating, you will continue to see those results for the REST OF YOUR LIFE! Let's be clear about a few things though: 80/20 doesn't mean eating perfectly Paleo 80 percent of the time and gorging on sugary, carb-loaded or chemical packed foods and beverages for the remaining 20 percent.

It means that after eating perfectly Paleo 80 percent of the time, if your budget and time constraints make the remaining 20 percent difficult to get perfect, you choose the next, most-Paleo option available to you. So if you eat free-range eggs most of the time, but this week you can only afford regular eggs, it doesn't mean that you reach for a bagel or cereal instead. It means that you get the regular eggs and maybe you add a dollop of grass-fed butter to them for an extra, more Paleo boost.

So, if sometimes you have to choose less-expensive and slightly less-Paleo options to make Paleo living work for you and your budget, don't sweat it. Doing Paleo 80/20 is literally a million times better than eating the standard American diet so many people are addicted to or even one of these low-fat, high-carb fad diets that doctors and nutritionists swear by. If you can manage 80/20 then be very proud of yourself, you WILL see the results your body and brain deserve.

4. **Learn to Shop Paleo:** While simply cutting out all of the overpriced, manufactured processed junk that makes

up the bulk of modern man's diet is enough to slice down your grocery bill, knowing how to shop for the right ingredients will make your Paleo meal plan a successful, delicious and inexpensive cinch!

Get Your Staples: As you know by now, the Paleo way of eating is grain-free but that doesn't mean that our ancient hunter ancestors lived off of just meat, meat and more meat. When it comes to Paleo staple, nutritious vegetables are the way to go, and the best part is that they are the cheapest items in your grocery store! Grab a whole bunch of leafy greens to round out your protein portions and you'll be shocked to see just how little you actually spend.

Head to the Great Outdoors: No, I don't mean you should go looking for food in the wilderness. I just mean that you should try your local outdoor farmer's market for the freshest, least expensive and most delectable array of fresh produce around. Farmer's markets are THE secret to shopping Paleo on a budget and getting the very best, most nutritious food possible.

Don't Sweat the Small Stuff: As you begin your Paleo journey, don't let the idea of shelling out big bucks for organic, naturally cultivated foods scare you off. While eating organic foods is definitely a great and healthy way to make sure we are living as closely to our ancient eating patterns as possible, it is not the be-all and end-all of the Paleo eating plan. If organic is too expensive for the majority of your meals, don't stress yourself out too much. Some organic produce is more important than other types. Steer clear of the most pesticide soaked types of produce(this can vary by area) and the crops most likely to be GMO and when it comes to the rest, just make sure that you are getting ample amounts of Paleo-friendly fruits and veggies and don't worry about focusing on just organic for the meantime. It is important to really get into Paleo-eating and allow your body to show you how much it truly needed this life change. After that, you can choose for yourself how much you're willing to spend on organic and grass-fed food products. And make no mistake, even if you aren't eating all organic, non-GMO and grass-fed items, as long as what you're eating is

Paleo, you're doing a whole lot more for your body than somebody regularly consuming grains and sugars(no matter how organic they may be).

Store Up Your Prey: Despite being called "uncivilized" societies, did you know that hunter-gatherers never wasted food like we do and were very clever at finding ingenious ways to preserve their food supplies to last them through lean times and harsh winters? With methods like fermenting and burying food, these hunters were able to keep their families and themselves fed and healthy to survive and thrive another year. Paleo eating is sustainable eating. How can you apply this to your own life? Well, don't worry, I'm not asking you to dig a hole in your backyard and ferment your freshly bought salmon steaks! What I mean by storing is making sure that you're thinking longer term rather than just "what should we have for dinner tonight?" This is where a lot of modern people go wrong today. We tend to think about food when we get hungry instead of planning ahead. When you look at your food as supplies and provisions that are there to feed AND nourish your healthy lifestyle, you'll stop wanting to reach for something fast, full of calories and "easy" and instead, map out a delicious plan to stay fit, slim and satisfied. Make a strategy and a budget and stick to it. Buy more pricey items like grass-fed beef and cage-free poultry meat in bulk and freeze them in individual labelled bags so that they can last for many months. When you need to get a quick meal together, it is as easy as grabbing an individual bag out of the freezer and defrosting! If you have other Paleo friends (we are a large community) consider buying in bulk together for truly HUGE savings. Make sure you store all of your fruits and vegetables properly, wrapping them in clean paper or cloth to keep them from getting frostbitten or wilted in your veggie section. Never waste leftovers. Simply store them well and use them for the next day's breakfast. Trust me, once you learn to store like a hunter, you'll find it easy to keep your monthly grocery bill well into the very low hundreds!

Make Smart Paleo Swaps: When people say Paleo food is expensive, it's because they think that a high protein, animal fat diet must be all fillet mignon and exotic fruits. That is simply not the case. There are literally tons of very smart Paleo swaps that you can make that will quickly cut down the cost and still deliver great Paleo nutrition and intense, amazing flavor.

Eggs: If you're looking for high-quality protein that delivers a nutritious, filling, versatile and tasty meal, look no further than that carton of eggs in the dairy section! When you think about it, a dozen eggs rarely costs more than a couple of bucks and yet you can make everything from Paleo omelets and scrambles to really gourmet fare like a no-crust, vegetable quiche or a cheesy, delicate French soufflé, just by cracking a couple!

Meat: When it comes to meat, don't feel that it has to be steak all the time. Instead, swap that steak for a delicious ground beef patty, cooked to perfection and garnished with full-fat butter. Also, don't let yourself be limited to the meat selection at your grocery store. Get to know your local butcher well and you will find that you can buy high-quality cuts for much less than in the supermarket when you purchase directly from the source.

Poultry: Eat the savory and nutrition-packed dark meat. Seriously, although white, lean chicken breast has gained a reputation as the "health" food of choice among the low-fat crowd, that's not what Paleo advocates. Eat the fattier, more flavorful dark meat for a fantastic source of rich nutrition and taste that will slim you down and bulk up your wallet at the same time!

Vegetables: Pre-washed, peeled and chopped veggies can be much more costly than whole ones at any grocery store. The answer: Do it yourself! Spending a few extra minutes washing, peeling and dicing your own vegetables at home will save you money and guarantee you the freshest, cleanest veggies possible. Also, keep in mind that vegetables lose their nutrients quickly after being exposed to air so those store bought ones may potentially have far less vitamins and minerals than the ones you prep at home.

Fruits: Always buying the freshest, most exotic fruits can get quite pricey. Instead, aim for making up a part of your fruit intake with delicious and healthy smoothies and sorbets made from whole, frozen berries. They are still packed with vitamins and nutrients and make for a budget-easy way to get the fruit you crave.

5. **Think Long Term:** Sure, grabbing a fast-food burger may seem like a simple, easy and cheap way to fill up for the moment, but if you look beyond the moment, you know that it has far-reaching and very expensive consequences. Food can be your medicine or it can be your poison, it can be your body's best friend or its very worst nightmare. The choice is yours. SO when you think about saving a couple of bucks and a few minutes of prep time by just ordering takeout or something quick from a drive-thru, don't forget that your body is being seriously damaged by each and every single poor eating choice you make and that one day, sooner rather than later, you will have to deal with the consequences. The consequences usually come in the form of a surprise injury or sudden illness, bringing with t huge medical bills or even just overall exhaustion, major weight gain and fatigue, making it impossible to do your job or live your life to the fullest. Don't forget that the average hospital stay can

easily average up to $20,000. That's 20,000 dollars for ONE single stay, because of ONE easily preventable health issue that the Paleo way of eating can help to eliminate! So when someone tells you that Paleo is expensive, remember that they are speaking from a place of inexperience: They either don't know or haven't learned how Paleo can be eaten on a budget and how it can help to prevent and heal so many costly medical issues and restore your energy, youthful vibrancy, health and appetite for life. How much is your health worth?

The Paleo way of eating and living can completely transform your health and life and the truth is that it doesn't have to cost more than sustaining an unhealthy fast-food habit or guzzling gallons of soft drinks. This book is packed with ideas and information that will help you to make your Paleo journey an easy, budget-friendly and delicious path for healing, rejuvenation, weight loss and longevity!

In the next chapter, we'll look at the one most important item you MUST stop poisoning your body and brain with right away!

Chapter 3:
The Bitter Secret about a Sweet Poison That is Ruining Your Health!

Our ancient ancestor, the Hunter, lived a hard life. Without a constant supply of food, adequate shelter or any medical care to speak of, he faced many challenges in trying to stay alive. And yet, even though we have plenty of food, housing and medical care, modern humans are facing a threat that is just as deadly if not deadlier than the ones faced by the Hunter. This threat is called sugar and it is literally killing millions of people around the world. You may think I am over-emphasizing the risk but consider this: Even as you read these words, sugar is busily causing terrifying and painful life-threatening conditions like metabolic syndrome, obesity, type 2 diabetes, cardiovascular diseases, strokes, autoimmune diseases from MS to lupus and neurodegenerative diseases like Parkinson's and Alzheimer's Disease. It is no wonder that sugar is now recognized by leading doctors and researchers as the single most deadly killer of our time. According to Dr. Robert Lustig, a renowned endocrinologist who has studied the link between sugar and ill-health, up to a whopping 75 % of all diseases afflicting Americans are now brought on by the SAD

(Standard American Diet) that sugar plays such a huge part in.

This means that the tens of millions of people who are suffering from the myriad of diseases brought on by consuming sugar are actually suffering needlessly! That's right. These conditions and diseases are completely preventable. How, you ask? The answer to that is very, very simple: Put down this book for a moment and walk over to your fridge and cupboards. Now, get rid of every last item containing refined sugar, from that big bag of cane sugar to all of those sodas, snacks, cereals and even canned goods, packed chockfull of sugar, dextrose, maltose, high fructose corn syrup and all of the other guises sugar hides its deadly poison in.

It really is that easy. If you do nothing else that is advised in this book to change your life and save yourself from the tidal wave of obesity, failing health and lethal diseases, taking this one simple action will SAVE YOUR LIFE! That's a big claim, but don't take my word for it. Take a look at the shocking evidence that backs up my statement, below:

Sugar and Diabetes: In a recent study, scientists looked at populations living in 17 different countries around the globe over a period of 10 years, in order to see whether different foods like meats, oils, fibers and sugar as well as social and economic factors like poverty, geography and aging had any kind of impact on the prevalence of type 2 diabetes. What these researchers found shocked everybody No type of food or socioeconomic factor had any kind of impact on the development of type 2 diabetes, except for one: Sugar. Out of all factors, only sugar availability was directly linked to the rapid rise of type 2 diabetes in populations around the world! This is as close as the medical and scientific world has ever come to admitting that yes, sugar consumption does lead to type 2 diabetes.

Sugar, High Fructose Corny Syrup and High Cholesterol: Several groundbreaking studies have shown a clear association between consumption of sugars like high fructose corn syrup and having higher levels of (bad) LDL cholesterol. These studies have shown that not only do your LDL levels go up when you consume sugar, but your risk of developing a variety of life-threatening cardiovascular diseases also goes up. I'm pretty sure that suddenly those helpings of sugar in your coffee cup aren't looking quite as enjoyable anymore.

Sugar Calories and Obesity: It has also been proven that all calories are not the same. When test subjects were made to replace nearly 30% of their daily total calories with calories from sugar-laden drinks, their weight shot right up, even though they were consuming the same amount of calories as usual. Nothing had changed except *where* their calories were coming from. What does this tell us? Calories from sugar are able to promote rapid weight gain, lead to obesity and even clog your heart's arteries in a way that non-sugar calories simply do not.

Sugar and Metabolic Syndrome: Metabolic syndrome, a collection of related diseases like type 2 diabetes, high blood pressure, high cholesterol with poor LDL to HDL balance, cardiovascular disease, non-alcoholic liver damage, a variety of cancers and dementias, is making major health headlines these days, as a newly emerging and dangerous threat. But if you thought this condition affected only overweight people, think again. Data now shows us that at least 40% of all normal weight people in the United States have developed one or all of the diseases and disorders that make up the metabolic syndrome spectrum. At the same time, a frightening 80% of all obese people manifest these diseases, too! This makes metabolic syndrome the most serious health emergency facing mankind today. So just what is behind its scary rise? That's right, sugar! Studies have proved that added sugars in foods and beverages are directly to blame for liver-contaminating, life-span shortening effects of this deadly syndrome! If you want to make sure that your body does not become yet another victim or statistic of this fast rising disease, kick sugar out of your life for good!

Sugar and Ageing: If you're like a lot of people, you have several expensive lotions and skin creams lining your bathroom shelves, in order to slow down or prevent the ageing process. But I've got news for you. If you are regularly consuming sugar in your food and beverages, then those lotions and creams won't do you an ounce of good. The reason I say this is because it is a fact that sugar consumption rapidly speeds up the ageing process, leaving you looking and feeling tired, ill and far older than your real age. It does this by acting on your proteins, lipids and your DNA to create permanent damage by literally binding fructose to them. Your skin becomes hard, rough, inflexible and dull. Instead of bouncing, it sags. Instead of lifting, it droops and quickly forms unsightly wrinkles. On the flip-side, try going without sugar for just a few days and then take a look in the mirror. The sudden health, glow and vitality of your complexion will do far more to convince you that you can put a stop to premature ageing by ditching the toxic white stuff, than all of the research in the world!

Sugar and Your Brain: "Sugar will rot your brain." How many times did you hear those words while growing up? Well, the facts are in and it is absolutely true. Even though it is impossible to say exactly how healthy the ancient brains of hunter-gatherers were, we do know that neurodegenerative diseases such as Parkinson's and Alzheimer's are not a "natural Part of ageing" as we are so often led to believe. We know this because, even though these diseases are highly common now in the WEST, they aren't in the rest of the world. If you look at other nations around the globe, you will find that actually, neurodegenerative disease and cognitive decline are very rare. On the other hand, here in the US and the West in general, rates of these neurodegenerative diseases are quickly skyrocketing, with even people as young as in their thirties presenting with signs of early onset dementia, for the first time ever in human history!

Why is this case? Well, if you look at the diets of developing nations where sugar is rarely eaten or drunk, you will quickly see that they also have correspondingly low rates of incidence for cognitive decline and dementias of any kind. When you look at the Western diet, however (especially the Standard American Diet), you can clearly see that it has been built on a dangerous foundation of added sugars. At the same time, you'll also notice that rates of cognitive decline and dementias of ALL kinds are rising right through the roof. This is not merely a hypothesis. Research shows us that consuming sugar leads to the disruption of your insulin levels. This then leads to a severe buildup of highly damaging amyloid proteins in your brai. Amyloid proteins are responsible for the development of dementia. Other studies also show that older people who ate diets that contained more sugars were much more likely to develop Alzheimer's or Parkinson's disease.

Anecdotally, people who go on the Paleo eating plan for the first time often report that removing sugar from their lives dramatically improves their long and short-term memory, their thinking skills, reaction time and ability to focus fully while carrying out difficult tasks. When we look at the lifestyles of our hunter-gatherer ancestors this makes perfect sense. The Hunter was never at risk of these mind-ruining and deadly diseases because he never had refined sugar available to him. Honey, his main source of sweetness, was a rare and very precious treat that was fiercely guarded by bees and therefore, not an easy, every day snack or staple, as so many sugary items have become for us today. As a result, the Hunter was able to stay sharp, alert and ultra-responsive to any changing circumstances or threats in his environment, allowing him to live to see another day in the dangerous wilderness that he roamed through. These days, as modern humans, we also face numerous dangers and challenges to our survival and it is absolutely certain that consuming sugar places a real drag on our mental processes today and may completely rob us of our ability to think at all tomorrow, if we continue to consume it.

Sugar and Cancer: Famed Nobel Laureate in medicine, Otto Warburg Ph.D., found out long ago that sugar is cancer's favorite food of choice. He showed how cancer cells were completely different from our healthy cells when it came to sources they used for energy. Cancer always rely on glucose(sugar) to feed them and guarantee their survival and high sugar consumption nourishes theses diseased cells, allowing them to spread, multiply and eventually, kill.

Sugar has been proven to be a major contributor to the increasing incidence of breast cancer in countries where a Western diet is widely consumed. Sugar has also been linked to a doubled and sometimes even tripled risk for pancreatic cancer, cancer of the biliary tract and liver cancer, among others. Starving cancer cells of their most loved food, sugar, can effectively force them to die off, because they cannot efficiently use any other food source for energy.

This list may seem frightening but the truth is, the diseases and disorders listed above are just a small sample of the many, many conditions that are caused by or exacerbated by sugar consumption. If you are convinced of sugar's deadly powers and you are ready to set yourself free from its addictive and destructive hold on you, checkout the list of items to eliminate and start you Paleo, sugar-free lifestyle today. You'll be saving your body, your brain and your life!

Remove The Following Sugars and Sugar Sources Completely from Your Diet:

- Table sugar

- All items containing added sugar, sucrose

- Anything containing:

- Sucrose

- Maltose

- Dextrose

- Dextran

- Dextrin

- Maltodextrin

- Fructose(Added)

- Glucose

- Galactose

- Lactose(Added)

- High Fructose Corn Syrup

- Glucose Solids

- Cane Juice

- Cane Juice Crystals

- Cane Juice (Dehydrated)

- Brown Sugar

- Barley malt

- Beet Sugar

- Corn Syrup

- Corn Syrup Solids

- Carob

- Malt Syrup

- Caramel

- Golden Syrup

- Turbinado Sugar

- Sorghum Syrup

- Diastase

- Ethyl Maltol

- Yellow Sugar

- Manitol

- Xylitol

Get rid of all packaged, processed foods (most of them are simply loaded with sugar) and all commercially prepared desserts, snacks and breakfast items. Make your own fresh sauces and condiments and do away with any store-bought ones because they are often a hidden sugar trap.

If you're wondering what you CAN use to add a little natural and healthy sweetness to your life, don't despair. There are some very good and completely natural, Paleo sweeteners out there that you can enjoy as part of an end of the week treat or a rare celebration:

Here is the list of fantastic tasting, natural, Paleo sweeteners to use once in a while:

- Organic Locally Sourced Raw Honey

- Pure Green Leaf Stevia or Pure Extract

- Dates(Especially Medjool Dates)

- Coconut Nectar

- Fruit juice (only fresh squeezed, real, organic

These five items are available in the wild and our hunter-gatherer ancestors could have accessed them sparingly, making these five sweeteners Paleo and perfectly OK for once in a while use.

Natural but Not as Fully Available In the Wild- Use Small Amounts Once in a Very Rare While

- Coconut sugar/crystals

- Maple syrup

- Palm sugar

These Sweeteners are Completely Artificial, Not Paleo and are Dangerous to Your Health, Never Use Them:

- Aspartame (***Nutra-Sweet, Equal***)

- Sucralose (***Spenda***)

- Tagatose (***PreSweet***

- Acesulfame K (***Sweet One***

- Stevia - white/bleached (***Truvia, Sun Crystals***)

- Saccarin (***Sweet'N Low***)

(If you're looking for more information on artificial sweeteners, make sure to check out the chapter on artificial additives and processed foods!)

Now that we've gotten this deadly "legal poison" out of the way, join me in the next chapter to find out why everyone is going against the grain and what this important Paleo move can do for your health, weight and energy!

See you there!

Chapter 4:
All Grains A Strain on the Brain.
Why Paleo Means Never Going Back to Grains!

If you are one of the millions of people who have been conscientiously following the "healthy eating" guidelines set out in the food pyramid and countless weight loss diets, by so-called experts, then you have probably struggling to understand why you are still experiencing bloating, exhaustion, unexplained and persistent weight gain as well as a general overall feeling of not being "well". Your fridge may be stocked with loads of heart-healthy, multi-grain, whole wheat foods and yet your cholesterol levels aren't looking very good and your low-fat, high grain diet seems not to be enough to keep your body from piling on the pounds. If this sounds familiar, then you are probably also disappointed, disillusioned and full of doubt when it comes to following yet another "diet". Well, don't despair because, as you will see, the Paleo way of eating is not simply another diet plan. It is a completely revolutionary way of resetting your body's clock to recapture the health, vigor, fitness, fat-burning and metabolism that human beings always naturally had. And in order to gain these amazing benefits, you have to do one very important thing: Ignore the experts! Yes, I said it! The USDA, the food pyramid, the doctors, nutritionists and the "diet gurus" everywhere who are trying to force you to deny your body's truth and instead, brainwash you into believing that eating a recommended 6-11 daily servings of something absolutely detrimental to human health is actually something good for you- ignore them all!

It may seem surprising to you that, when it comes to grains, the Paleo way of eating goes against the conventional advice of doctors and nutritionists but think about it: How many millions of people (yourself included) have tried to eat all of the grains prescribed as healthy by these same doctors and nutritionists? And how many of those millions of people end up feeling sicker and more tired, looking older and more bloated, and suffering with everything from obesity to depression, autoimmune disorders to dementia? So when it come s to your own life, you've got to take back control and refuse to let the outdated and completely misleading nutritional guidelines of the food pyramid and the nutritionists lead you to physical and emotional pain, exhaustion and the total destruction of your mind and body. To win back your valuable health, you've got to go against the grain!

List of Grains to Eliminate From Your Diet:

- Amaranth

- Barley

- Brown rice

- Brown rice bread

- Brown rice tortilla

- Buckwheat

- Kamut

- Bulgur

- Farro

- Emmer

- Einkorn

- Flaxseed

- Millet

- Oats

- Oat bread

- Oatmeal

- Popcorn

- Whole wheat cereal

- Muesli

- Rolled oats

- Quinoa(not a "real" grain but nonetheless, a non-Paleo grain-like substance)

- Rye (Whole or Not)

- Sorghum

- Spelt

- Teff

- Triticale

- Wheat berries

- Whole grain cornmeal

You may be wondering, just what it is about grains that can cause such damage to the human body and brain Well, because grains affect us negatively on so many levels , there are many answers to that question. Let's look at some of them:

Diseases: We have been told for a very long time by scientists that disease is coded into human DNA and that our genes are the number one decider of whether we will get sick or not and what kind of diseases we may develop in the future. That simply is not true. Diseases are not inscribed in our destiny. Instead, it is our lifestyle choices that are the deciding factors between health and illness. Where do grains fit in to all of this? Grains cause diseases like gasoline fuels fires. We may eat them for many years without ever really realizing how we are dragging our bodies and minds to the very edge of destruction and then one day, when we tip over the edge, suddenly we find our health going up in flames.

Here are some of the top ways that grain consumption can totally throw off our bodies' natural balance, health and metabolism:

Grains Equal a Dangerous Carbohydrate Rush: Refined sugars aren't the only substance s we should be worried about. When it comes to triggering a speedy rise in our insulin levels, grains can be just as bad. Because grains are simple sugars, they are very rapidly and easily broken down into sugar. The resulting rise in our blood glucose levels signals the start of a crazy insulin rollercoaster in our bodies' that can leave us with permanent nerve, tissue and organ damage. When we eat the "recommended" diet of heaps upon heaps of grains, we often feel completely bone tired.

That is because all of those grains are taking their toll on our insulin levels, keeping them impossibly high for longer and longer periods, creating a truly frightening situation for our bodies and brains. Modern man is now facing an unprecedented epidemic of frequently elevated insulin levels. Normally, this hormone's primary job is to manage levels of sugar in your blood. When glucose levels stay too elevated for too long, the body is faced with an onslaught and as a result, develop a resistance to insulin. At this stage, even more insulin is produced in order to flood your cells with and the insulin rush plus insulin resistance pattern begins to emerge. When this happens metabolic syndrome, a syndrome with massive implications for the future health of mankind, begins to take place.

Constantly elevated levels of insulin are standing in the way of most Americans desire to lose weight because high insulin levels prevent the body from being able to burn off the fat, instead turning the body's attention to making the surplus of glucose in the blood into your main energy source. Whatever is left unused at the end of this process is quickly packed away on your body as stubborn fat. This stubborn fat then rapidly turns into a particularly difficult to lose store of stomach blubber and as we all know, those excessive tires of abdominal fat, called visceral fat, are the single most serious health threat of our time, bringing us face to face with the risk of heart attacks and strokes, aneurysms, type 2 diabetes –led organ death, vicious inflammation and breathing disorders such as emphysema. This is why we say those friendly USDA guidelines regarding the wonderful benefits of grains are some of the most deadly pieces of health advice you can take.

Aside from an insane carbohydrate load, grains also saddle the human digestive system with another very serious problem, anti-nutrients.

Phytates: Phytates are found in grains and their damaging effect on the human body comes from the way they bind themselves to the minerals such as calcium, iron, zinc, magnesium and copper in our food, preventing us from being able to absorb and utilize these minerals for our health and well-being. Even when eating a diet that is very rich in mineral content, you can end up with severe nutritional deficiencies. This makes those nutritional arguments that you should eat plenty of grains for their "healthy mineral content" completely pointless, because every time you eat a supposedly mineral-rich slice of whole wheat bread for instance, the phytates contained in that bread have basically stolen your desired mineral supply from you. A Paleo diet that is full of proteins, fats, vegetables, seeds, fruits and nuts can provide you with nutrients you can EASILY and FULLY use, unlike grain-based diets that strip away their "benefits" before you even get a chance to absorb them! (Note: Phytates are also found in much lower and less harmful amounts in nuts and seeds which are Paleo approved. To enjoy your nuts and seeds and still harness all of the nutrition you need, try soaking them in either water, a lemon and water mix or pure yogurt. This will "digest" the phytates for you so that your body doesn't have to do the hard work.

Lectins: Lectins are found in all grains and are extremely dense, tough and tiny, making them an absolute nightmare for the human digestive system. Leptins destroy the intestinal walls by allowing openings to be made in them and thus, allowing for the development of leaky gut disorder. They damage the gut lining which leads to leaky gut and other disorders. When leaky gut syndrome strikes, you know that autoimmune diseases and disorders are not far behind, as these openings in the intestinal wall lining can only mean that potentially toxic, undigested foods, bacteria and other harmful materials can easily slip out of the intestines through these holes, entering your blood and crossing the blood/brain barrier and without further ado, you can find yourself in a scary autoimmune cycle, facing down your own immune system and hoping that you will not destroy your own body. Lectins are impossible to destroy with heat so even if you cook them thoroughly, they will still remain tough and inedible. In addition to all of this, lectin actually suppresses your appetite control system, leaving you always feeling ravenous, constantly snacking and never full! Also, all members of the grass family contain very high amounts of lectin so it is very important to steer clear of wheats, wheat grass and other grass grains in particular. When our bodies come into contact with lectins, after a few run-ins, our immune systems react with ferocity, fighting by creating powerful antibodies to target and neutralize the foreign threat. However, what happens when your own tissue looks so similar to the lectins your body is fighting? The result is usually the large scale destruction of your own tissue, with your immune system going rogue and leaving you damaged, ailing and perhaps even in danger of losing organ function.

Gluten: Now for the third and perhaps, the very worst of the deadly grain quartet, gluten. Gluten is a difficult to breakdown protein that can be found in many commonly eaten grains such as:

- White Flour

- Whole Wheat Flour

- Durum Wheat

- Semolina

- Spelt

- Wheat Germ

- Wheat Bran

- Graham Flour

- Triticale

- Kamut

Gluten is commonly found in these food items as well:

- Cereal

- Crackers

- Sodas

- Beer

- Oats (see the section on oats below)

- Gravy

- Dressings

- Sauces

- Couscous

- Bread

- Flour Tortillas

- Pasta

- Cakes

- Muffins

- Pastries

Gluten is now found in much higher amounts within today's modern grains, with levels reaching 80 %, than ever existed in ancient grains. All gluten containing substances are capable of creating a state called agglutination, a reaction that causes suspended particles to coagulate in big clumps. What does this do to our bodies?

- Gluten-led agglutination causes the creation of pro-inflammatory chemicals, in response to what the body perceives as a major injury.

- Gluten destroys the protective covering over neurons, and stops nerve growth factor from helping neurons to live.

- Gluten acts on the body and brain like any viruses and research shows that the body views it as just such a dangerous invader, triggering a damaging response.

- Gluten forces the clumping of blood platelets, disrupting their normal functions.

The gliadin content in today's wheat also causes inflammatory cytokine activity that leads to numerous tiny holes being drilled into the important intestinal wall lining, resulting in a nasty case of leaky got (gut permeability). Zonulin, a protein molecule produced when we eat gluten, also contributes to leaky gut by loosening the usually tight junctions within the intestinal cell walls. This permeability opens up the gut, allowing undigested, partially digested and toxic food and other particles, like bacteria to slip into the bloodstream where they cause havoc. This in turn leads to diseases and disorders such as autoimmune disorders like chronic fatigue syndrome, rheumatoid arthritis, multiple sclerosis, lupus, chronic fatigue syndrome, fibromyalgia, inflammatory bowel disease (ulcerative colitis) and asthma. Up to a third of the adult population has lab visible amounts of anti-gliadin within their stools.

All Grains a Strain on Your Brain!

These anti-gliadin antibodies are the result of your body's protective response to the "invader" gluten and are a clear indication of inflammation. In the same way as it causes leaky gut, gluten can also cause leaky brain syndrome or increased permeability of the vital blood brain barrier. When gluten inflames the brain, it forces openings in what is a usually closed barrier, allowing numerous harmful food antigens and even bacterial pathogens to flood into the brain, causing disease, loss of cognitive abilities, loss of memory, anger, depression, confusion, and even certain manifestations of mental illness. The symptoms of brain fog and emotional disturbance are only sign posts, signaling that the constant inflammation your brain is being subjected to through gluten or grain consumption will eventually lead to a terrifying and painful neurodegenerative disease like Parkinson's , Alzheimer's disease or dementia. All grains effectively light your brain on fire and let it slowly burn its way down to the very end, causing untold suffering and much invisible damage before the results are clear. If that sounds scary, it's because it is. Our brains are our most important organs and safeguarding them has to be a priority for the survival minded human. Without a well- protected and well-functioning brain, you quickly go from being the predator to being the prey!

Protease Inhibitors: Aside from the gluten, lectin, phytates and elevated insulin response, grains also contain yet another dangerous stumbling block that trips up anybody trying to find the road to good health by including them into their diet. These stumbling blocks are protease inhibitors and they are the body's equivalent of gasoline being poured on a raging wildfire! When you consume grains of any kind, protease inhibitors slow down or stop proper digestion of protein within your gut. Not only does this mean you have an even harder time dealing with lectins, but it also means you can't digest those very beneficial proteins you're getting from nutrient rich sources. This basically boils down to one sad fact: It doesn't matter how much high quality, fantastic protein you're gulping down, protease inhibitors will not allow you to use them. So if you are eating rains, you may just as well NOT spend your money on buying expensive lean chicken breast, organic lamb meat or pastured beef, because in the end. Your body doesn't see an ounce of the benefits, so long as protease inhibitors are doing their dastardly work.

Paleo Alternatives to Grains: How to Make You No- Grain Diet Work For Your Body and Your Budget!

Just because you've gone Paleo does not mean you've suddenly become immune to the once in a rare while cravings for certain baked products. But when you're faced with that craving, does this automatically mean you should just go for the cake, cookies or pizza in front of you? Absolutely not, especially when there are some very Paleo ways to circumvent those cravings and still stay on track, healthy and happy. Here are some awesome and money saving Paleo non-grain tips to try put today!

On rare occasions, go for almond or coconut flours: Yes, these flours tend to be a bit pricey but as long as you use them on only the rarest of occasions, you should be good to go. One way to make the best of these flours without busting your budget is to use them in mousses and other very low-flour requirement recipes, allowing you to use just a little of these flours and still get your once in blue moon, Paleo dessert fix!

Learn to soak nuts and seeds, sprout them and turn them into your very own homemade flours: Almond and coconut flours can be expensive and can get repetitive if you only use the two, so instead, learn to make your own nut and seed flours.

Soaking your nuts and seeds before use will allow you to eliminate any unpleasant and potentially harmful enzyme inhibitors present in them. Additionally soaking allows us ot properly digest and utilize the nuts and seeds by helping the release of phytates, a potential risk in nuts and seeds (although occurring in much lower amounts within them than within grains) that could prevent the correct absorption of vital minerals.

How to soak your nuts and seeds:

1. Start with raw nuts or raw seeds.

2. Place the nuts or seeds in a large bowl (Ensure that it is large enough to handle

any swelling in size that could occur) and pour filtered water over them until they are fully covered.

3. Allow them to soak in the bowl overnight.

4. Remove the water from the bowl, leaving the nuts or seeds behind.

5. Your nuts or seeds are now cleared of excessive amounts of anti-nutrients and enzyme inhibitors, allowing you to either use them immediately or keep them in a closed container in the fridge for a couple of days.

You may also choose to sprout your nuts and seeds. Sprouting is an entirely natural process that can ramp up levels of valuable nutrition within your nuts or seeds.

How to Sprout Your Nuts or Seeds:

1. Start with completely raw nuts or seeds that have already been soaked.

2. Place them on a large plate and arrange them so that they each have a little room between them.

3. Cover the nuts or seeds loosely with either a piece of unbleached muslin or a cheese cloth

4. Make sure that your rinse twice daily

5. When sprouting begins, it will be indicated by the appearance of a small white "tail-like" growth on the narrow side of the nuts or seeds

6. At this point you can use your nuts and seeds immediately or place in a sealed container in the fridge instead.

Top Tip: Use these soaked or sprouted nuts and seeds to make yourself a seriously delicious, nutrient rich and very inexpensive Paleo homemade granola. Dry your nuts and seeds thoroughly and toss them in the oven or dehydrator along with a good coating of raw, pure honey, a few drops of stevia, a pinch of nutmeg, cloves and cinnamon as well as bit of salt to season!

As soon as you get rid of the grains in your life, you will begin to feel and look more like you were always intended to, strong, healthy lean, happy and alert. You'll enjoy the anti-inflammatory benefits of having a glowing, youthful complexion, a light, agile and muscled body, an extra boost in your step, a continual natural energy and a quick thinking mind that won't let you down! No matter how much you adore donuts or live off of sugary cereals, trust me, nothing made of grains can ever taste as good as finally claiming victory over your health, weight gain and emotional as well as cognitive challenges, once and for all! You owe yourself a chance to see the amazing unfulfilled potential that grains have been keeping your from unleashing for many years. That's why I'm ending this chapter with a challenge: Try going absolutely grain free for 1 month. Within that time, do not consume any drink, food or snack with grains of any kind in it. Certainly, after the first addiction withdrawal pangs, you will find yourself looking and feeling lighter, healthier, more vibrant and vital than ever before. And I guarantee that once you've experienced your body and brain without grains, you'll get rid of this unhealthy strain for good!

Chapter 5:
The Paleo Dairy Question: To Milk or Not to Milk?

While the Paleo way of eating definitely has some very firm ground rules and no-go areas (for example: No sugar and absolutely no grains!) when it comes to the matter of whether or not to consume dairy products, there is a certain amount of room for personal opinion and choice. This is because dairy is capable of being a very nutritionally rich source of important animal proteins and fats that can add to your health and weight loss success on a paleo eating plan, provided that you are able to tolerate dairy. The question of whether or not dairy is for you can only really be properly answered by doing a simple elimination test and following this up with a gradual reintroduction process. I've included an easy step by step plan to help you carry out this process by yourself at home and definitively figure out if dairy products deserve a place at you Paleo table. Before we get to the elimination and reintroduction process, however, let's take a look at the different positive and negative aspects of dairy:

Is dairy truly Paleo? : Did early hunter-gatherer societies have access to animal dairy? The simple answer to this is no. Because our hunter-gatherer ancestors did not keep and domesticate animals, they would have had little opportunity to obtain milk from an animal source. As you can imagine it would have been rather difficult and dangerous to try to milk wild undomesticated and free roaming animals, so no, early hunter-gatherers were not really milk drinkers in the sense that we mean today. However, this does not automatically translate into the idea that human beings were never meant to consume milk. In fact, dairy (in the form of nutrient rich breast milk) is the highly beneficial first food of all human beings and despite the modern shift towards artificial milk formula as a substitute, maternal milk remains the very best possible source of initial nutrition for humans as we start out life. Research into breast milk has found that it contains a truly astounding amount of beneficial nutrients, proteins and saturated fats. It is also rich in good, helpful bacteria, essential fatty acids and has been directly linked to proper and healthy physical and mental development in the young. For this reason alone, we know that the human body can utilize milk in an effective and highly positive way.

Opponents of including milk on a paleo diet point out that if our ancient hunter ancestors weren't milking wild wildebeests, then we shouldn't be swilling down animal dairy in any form. My answer to this is quite clear cut: If we take that approach then there is a long list of healthy and important foods on the Paleo eating plan including such items as coconut oil and coconut milk, smoothies, almond flour, nut butters and other foods, that were definitely not available to our Paleo ancestors in the same form as we use and enjoy them today.

That does not mean that they are automatically not Paleo and that certainly does not take away from their very real health value to humans. In the case of dairy many Paleo/Primal adherents will agree that it is the WAY you consume it and not the inherent nature of dairy itself that makes the biggest impact on whether dairy adds to or detracts from your Paleo eating plan.

Dairy and Beneficial Bacteria: Something to really look at when considering the dairy question is the abundance of good bacteria it can provide. With the rise of modern autoimmune diseases and disorders, the topic of probiotic use has become a major talking point in the healthy eating world. This is because we now know that the over processed, over sterilized and nutritionally dead character of the foods we humans tend to eat today has drastically upset the delicate balance of our gut flora, rendering us prone to illness. When our gut bacteria is destroyed, human health suffers in a myriad of surprising ways, from the development of seasonal and food allergies to autoimmune disorders, depression, chronic inflammation leading to permanent tissue damage and even organ failure. Probiotics can be used to successfully repopulate the gut with good bacteria and help to diminish the overgrowth of harmful bad bacteria, preventing and healing damage and disease. Dairy products can be used as very efficient probiotics, provided that they are in a raw form. They do their best probiotic work when they have first been fermented into a variety of beneficial dairy foods and beverages such as kefir, live active yogurt, fermented buttermilk and certain cheeses.

Another benefit of dairy can be found in its high animal fat content, making it a deeply satiating and actually very paleo item to consume. Research has shown us that fatty dairy products can have an appetite reducing and weight loss enhancing effect on your body, when consumed regularly. Although previous erroneous ideas about the supposed "dangers" of consuming fatty dairy products have no real scientific basis, the resulting use of low-fat dairy products has been largely to blame for the negative reputation dairy sometimes has. However, recent and convincing research proves that there is direct like between consuming MORE dairy fat and having IMPROVED health markers. Contrary to the conventional medical myths that are only just now being debunked, consuming full-fat dairy does not lead to an increased incidence of cardiovascular disease and is actually associated with long term heart health. Fermented full-fat dairy has also been shown to be beneficial in preventing the development of cardiovascular disease. Despite dairy's reputation as an insulin spiking food item, tests actually show that when obese research subjects up their consumption of dairy, it results in lowered insulin resistance and decreased risk of diabetes development. Other amazing benefits of dairy include everything from lowered blood pressure to the elimination of stored and stubborn stomach fat, a regulated appetite as well as improved cholesterol levels and lipid profile. In yet more studies, increased intake of full fat cheese containing high levels of vitamin K2 led to decreased risk of developing a wide range of deadly cancers.

Dairy fat is naturally the richest and most complex of all types of fat, consisting of more than 400 different types of positive fatty acids like CLA or Conjugated Linoleic Acid, a super healthy fat that, when consumed from natural sources such as cheese, is able to significantly lower inflammation and eliminate the risk of cardiovascular complications. Butyric acid, another positive fat found in dairy, can even alleviate and heal inflammatory conditions like Crohn's disease. Milk Fat Globule Membrane (or MFGM, for short) found in high amounts in fatty dairy items, can also heal hypertension and improve your overall lipid profile.

Now that we've taken a look at the benefits of dairy, let's examine the potential dangers and challenges of dairy consumption and how to decide what's best for your body:

Lactose Intolerance: The most commonly reported negative effect in relation to dairy consumption is difficulty digesting milk's lactose content. Lactose intolerance occurs when a person is have sufficient production of an enzyme called lactase, that is necessary in order to break down the lactose sugars inherent in milk and milk products . The result is that when a lactose intolerant person consumes these dairy products, they are unable to digest the lactose and are often left suffering from side effects like bloating, indigestion, pain, muscle and joint aches, inflammation, acne, brain fog, mood swings and weight gain.

Sensitivity to Casein: Casein is a major protein found in milk (particularly cow's milk) and has been linked to negative symptoms similar to the kinds of symptoms experienced in cases of gluten intolerance. These include migraines, weight gain, nerve damage, ataxia, apraxia, memory loss, cloudy thinking, mouth ulcers, learning and cognitive impairment and bowel problems including constipation, excess mucus and diarrhea.

Those who claim that milk is unnatural to the human body often cite its casein content. However, they overlook the fact that human breastmilk contains a large amount of casein and is well tolerated by and even nourishing to humans today, just as it was to our ancient ancestors. This clearly shows us that casein is not the root of the problem. Instead, recent research is shedding light on the fact that casein may not be the true culprit behind all of these severe reactions and that a serious case of gut dysbiosis, a common problem, may actually be to blame for modern humans' sensitivity to casein. If you are suffering from a suspected case of casein sensitivity, you may actually be the victim of an inflamed gut that is causing undigested casein particles to float out of your stomach lining and into your blood stream, where they can then set off the series of unpleasant reactions listed above.

A Note on Healing Casein Sensitivity: The best way to deal with this issue is to put yourself on a strictly Paleo diet and eliminate all inflammatory irritants (such as sugars, grains and nightshade vegetables like tomatoes, eggplants and peppers) from your eating plans and consume large amounts of pure homemade beef and chicken bone broth. In many cases, once the irritants have been removed from your diet, the healing bone broths can then help to mend the "open wounds" in your intestinal lining, allowing you to consume casein-containing milk and other dairy products without an adverse reaction, within just a few weeks.

Important Factors to Consider with Dairy Consumption:

Pasteurization: This is the most important factor (after figuring out your personal tolerance or allergy risk) when deciding whether or not to consume a certain dairy product. If the dairy product you are considering adding to your meal is not pasteurized, then you will have a much lower chance of suffering any ill effects from consuming it and you will also benefit more fully from the nutrients that are found in non-pasteurized milk products. What about pasteurized milk products? I'd like to answer this very definitively so you can be really clear about the matter: I do not and cannot recommend the consumption of pasteurized milk or any products made from pasteurized to anyone, whether they are on the Paleo eating plan or not. This is because pasteurization is a completely man-made and damaging process that destroys the intrinsic goodness of real, raw milk, turning it into a dangerous substance instead of the healthy, nutritious food source that it is.

Pasteurization basically "kills" milk, stripping it of all its useful properties and making it very difficult to digest for the average human. One of the ways that it does this is by totally destroying the important enzymes within milk that are meant to help our bodies' digest it. At the same time, pasteurization also eliminates essential vitamins found in milk such as vitamin A , vitamin B6 , vitamin B12 and vitamin C. During the pasteurization process, milk's normally useful proteins are warped into unrecognizable amino acid structures and when our bodies are confronted with these strange structures, it often reacts to what it sees as a distinctly foreign substance by triggering a variety of illnesses and allergies. And the horrors of pasteurization don't stop there, either. Milk that has been pasteurized has also been completely robbed of its abundant supply of beneficial bacteria. These probiotic bacteria are able to promote gut health by exerting a positive healing, disease- fighting and anti-pathogenic effect on the gut environment. Once they are wiped out by the harsh pasteurization process, you are left with a substance falsely labelled "milk" that is actually no longer like real milk at all. Instead, it is a dangerous, unnatural liquid that provokes pathogenic overgrowth and fuels inflammation, leading to leaky gut syndrome, a precursor to numerous, difficult to treat health issues.

There is nothing natural, instinctive or nourishing about the pasteurization process and there is nothing Paleo about pasteurized milk. So when you hear that milk could potentially be a healthy part of your Paleo diet, please remember that this refers to real, raw milk.

Raw Milk: The most optimal way to consume dairy without the dangerous and destructive effects of pasteurization is to always make sure that your milk and milk products have never been pasteurized and are completely raw. Raw milk is milk in its most natural state and thus, is the type of milk best recognized, tolerated and utilized by our bodies.

The benefits of raw milk include:

Nutrition: Raw milk contains all of the nutrients that are destroyed by the pasteurization process. Studies show that pasteurization eliminates milks supply of copper, iron and manganese and the FDA warns that pasteurization also ruins the supply of vitamin C in milk, while the sterilization process makes milk's vitamin B6 supply unusable. Pasteurization also destroys milk's store of beta-lactoglobulin, a fragile protein that is easily ruined by heat. Beta-lactoglobulin is useful in helping your intestines to absorb and utilize vitamin A and is found in abundance in raw, non-pasteurized milk. Raw milk is able to preserve all of these nutrients and allow you to benefit from them, every time you take a sip.

Lack of Intolerance: A survey of several hundred families suffering from lactose intolerance and casein sensitivity showed that once these individuals switched from drinking pasteurized milk to only consuming raw milk, the lactose intolerance and all accompanying symptoms VANISHED!

Taste: Those who have made the switch from dead pasteurized milk to fresh raw milk say that raw milk has a much more wholesome, delicious, real and pure taste. It is creamier, richer and almost palatably more nutritious than the flat, watery substance now called pasteurized "milk".

Allergy protection an Immune System Moderation: Large amounts of epidemiological evidence from European studies prove that early childhood consumption of raw milk can have a protective effect against allergies and asthma, while also preventing immune-led disorders. Anecdotal evidence proves that raw milk consumption has also been linked to a decrease of allergic symptoms and an improvement in autoimmune disease symptoms in adults who begin drinking raw milk.

In light of its superior nutrient content, damage-preventative and healing powers and disease fighting properties, raw milk is far better than pasteurized milk. While personal choice is everything when it comes to deciding whether or not to include dairy on your Pale eating plan, I would like to advise you to only include dairy if it will be raw. It is far better to get no milk at all than to drink the poison that is pasteurized milk, these days!

Grass-fed: The best milk comes from cows that have been allowed to graze for grass rather than being forced fed an inappropriate grains diet.

Cows that are grain-fed produce milk and meat that are both very high in omega 6 fatty acids, to the detriment of the desirable omega 3 fatty acids that your body needs.

Animal Type: When it comes to how well you tolerate milk and can reap its rewards, the answer may depend on the livestock species or breed that your milk and milk products come from. These days, many people prefer to get their milk supply from milking goats or even sheep because their milk provides low casein and less irritation. Another tip to help with any lactose intolerance you may experience is to try switching to an older breed of cow. In the US and most of North America, most cows are type A1, a newer breed of cows that experienced a mutation nearly 5000 years ago. These types of cows provide large amounts of milk but also bring large amounts of pain, inflammation, sinus allergies with them, due to levels of the dangerous opiate BCM7.

A2 cow breeds from Africa and Asia are way older than the kind in the US and North America in general, and their milk, since it is more "familiar" to your body (without BCM7), can be tolerated without problems, in the majority of cases.

Making Your Paleo Dairy Delights Affordable: Some people argue that raw milk is simply way too expensive when compared to conventional pasteurized milk, but the truth is ONLY raw milk IS milk and that the milky pasteurized substance called "milk" is actually a ridiculous impersonation of the full fat , creamy , healthy raw milk.

But all of this only matters if you can actually afford to switch from the pasteurized stuff to the nourishing raw milk, right? So here are some tips to help make your Paleo dairy habit an inexpensive treat:

Deal Directly With The Farmer: Forget shops (raw milk is not allowed to be retailed in most states, anyway) and head straight to your nearest raw milk producing dairy farm. Negotiating with the owners for a good price can help you to get top of the line raw milk at rock-bottom prices. Bring your own containers, for a further discount.

Buy Herd Shares; If you live in a state where raw milk sales are illegal (due to often overstated and misguided concerns) or you simply want to get the best bang for your buck, purchase a local herd share in grass-fed livestock and get your portion of very affordable, high quality, raw milk!

Waste not, Want not: This tip applies to the proper storage of your delicious Paleo dairy loot. Once you've bought your milk for a great price, it is important to put a portion away for days when you will need it. Making ice cubes out of the creamy milk is one great and effective way of keeping your raw milk for longer. When you require some milk, your simply remove as many raw milk cubes as need and pop the tray back into the freezer. Proper storage is absolutely necessary because it allows you to buy in large amounts, snaring yourself a discount and keeping your raw milk fresh and easily available for longer.

Raw milk can help to ease everything from allergies to eczema and prevent heart disease, weight gain, depression and even cancer. Follow the tips above to get the very best and most affordable raw milk benefits possible for your body and mind!

How to Determine Your Level of Dairy Tolerance:

IMPORTANT: First, please note that if you have a dairy ALLERGY or have ever had a

serious to severe reaction to consuming dairy before, you should NOT try an at home elimination and reintroduction test. Instead, speak with your doctor and find out how best to get a safe medical diagnosis for your symptoms!

Step 1: Elimination: remove all dairy products from your diet. This includes all milk, cheese, butter, yogurt, kefir, sour cream, buttermilk and cream.

Step 2: Time: Keep this elimination period up for a minimum of 30 days. This will give you the time necessary to really see how your body reacts to life without dairy and give your body a chance to heal from any previous dairy –led inflammation, so that you get the clearest results possible.

Step 3: Re-introduction: After the dairy free 30 days, slowly add each eliminated dairy item back into your diet, one at a time.

Step 4: Make Notes: Keep detailed notes about how you felt without diary and then how you felt as each dairy item was reintroduced. This will help you pinpoint whether you have a real intolerance to dairy or you are more tolerant of certain kinds f dairy products or amounts than others.

Raw milk and dairy products made from this raw milk can help to ease everything from allergies to eczema and prevent heart disease, weight gain, depression and even cancer. Follow the tips above to get the very best and most affordable Paleo raw milk benefits possible for your body and mind!

Chapter 6:
Understanding Vegetables the Paleo Way

While the Paleo way of eating's guidelines differ widely on many points from the advice of conventional "nutrition experts", the Paleo diet shares the view that vegetables can be a very potent form of nourishment and healing. While Paleo has a healthy respect for vegetables, one major difference you will see as you join this movement is that Paleo eaters do not put vegetables on a special pedestal, above all other forms of food. Many fad diets tell people to make vegetables their number one source of nutrition. They advise that more than half a person's plate should be loaded with nothing but lightly cooked veggies and that doing this will somehow spur on weight loss and health while still keeping hunger at bay. If you have ever tried one of these "healthy eating plans", you know that the results are not at all as advertised: You often end up hungry, cranky, losing only very little weight or even gaining more weight than you started with and feeling tired, bloated and sick.

That is NOT what Paleo is about. Instead, Paleo is all about eating in a naturally beneficial way that follows as closely as possible, the healing, revitalizing and nourishing eating patterns that the human body has always and will always desire to follow. Paleo definitely has a special place for vegetables but, have no fear, that place is NOT on over half of your plate! Rather, vegetables are a part of (not most of) a healthful eating plan that also includes plenty of rich, satisfying and delicious proteins and fats, so that you are never left hungry, tired or cranky and so that, far from gaining weight, you actually lose weight so quickly that it is almost immediately noticeable. And most of all, Paleo is about sustaining these amazing results. If you lose weight on the Paleo eating plan, rest assured that it will not be for a week or a month. Instead, as long as you mostly follow this ancient and instinctive way of eating (easy to do, since it is so delicious and satiating!) you will have amazing weight loss, energy and health results for LIFE! And the best part is, you don't have to try to turn into a human rabbit and only live off of raw lettuce to obtain and maintain these results. If this sounds good, then let's take a look at the role that vegetables played in our ancestral diets and how to follow that in our diets today.

Our ancient hunter-gatherer ancestors were not settled farmers. They got their nutrition from the wild environment around them and were always sure to choose foods that required very little

cooking and were found in a relatively ready-to –
eat state. This also applies to vegetables. The
Hunter may have found many types of wild
vegetables growing freely in the forests or
wilderness and these he would have been able to
eat just as they were.

Today, the Paleo way of eating stresses the
importance of eating a good amount of certain
Paleo-friendly vegetables while also stressing the
necessity of avoiding certain vegetables that are
not a historic or healthy part of our human diets
and can instead, pose serious digestive problems
to the body.

Let's look at the best vegetables to make up the
largest part of your veggie portions on a Paleo
eating plan:

Wild leafy greens that were the forerunners of
the kale, spinach and other greens that we
consume today made up the bulk of the Hunter's
vegetable diet. He would rely on these to provide
a supplementary source of energy to the animal
fat and protein he was consuming. While almost
all vegetables (non-starchy or low-starch ones, in
particular) can make a healthy contribution to
our diets, these vegetables should be staples on
your Paleo eating plan:

Spinach- Dark, leafy green, low in calories, high in minerals, nutrients and antioxidants and extremely affordable, as well as filling. Make a lightly blanched spinach salad a common addition to your meaty Paleo main dishes!

Kale – Kale is also as nutrient-rich as spinach, and with its heavier, denser nature, it is even more filling than spinach and other greens. Kale is packed with a large quantity of phytonutrients that are capable of fending off cancer and warding off damage caused by free radicals! It

Dandelion Greens-These excellent green forage plants (that can be found in stores, too!) make for a healthy, low-cost, high nutrient addition to your Paleo plate and they are fantastic as a way of detoxing from modern da chemicals because of their highly diuretic and detoxifying properties.

Collard Greens – Collard greens are sturdy, heavily flavored and can sand up well to slow cooking and braising methods. They are also highly economical and just as nutrient-dense as other greens like kale and spinach. Make them a part of your Paleo meals and warm salads.

Seaweed- Often called the spinach of the sea, seaweed was a major component of the ancient hunter-gatherers who dwelled near oceans. It can provide a surprising amount of nutrition (some excellent quality iodine content, for healthy thyroid function) and is very low in calories.

Cucumber – Cucumbers are loaded with good water content and can help you to stay hydrated when added to a salad or even to your drinking water, for a fresh tasting, super-hydrating thirst quencher.

Mushrooms – Mushrooms are THE Paleo mainstay as hunter-gatherers were able to easily forage them as an addition to their meals. Higher in protein than most non-animal products, mushrooms also contain literally thousands of as yet not-fully studied compounds that somehow seem to aid health. Some effects that have been proved however are hormone-regulation, anti-cancerous properties and low-calorie, nutrient-density, so make sure you add them to your mains and sides, for real hunter-gatherer nutrition!

Please Note: Our ancestors were "professional" hunters and gatherers and even they occasionally picked and ate dangerous mushrooms by accident. Please do NOT forage for your own

mushrooms. Instead, purchase them from trusted stores because even one poisonous mushroom could be deadly and is NOT worth the risk!

Other Vegetables: Most vegetables including beets, carrots, various onions, lettuce of all kinds, peppers, tomatoes and eggplants (if you are not allergic to nightshades or on the autoimmune Paleo protocol) cruciferous vegetables and other greens, are all Paleo and can be enjoyed in large amounts, as long as you are including ample amounts of the vegetables listed above in the preferred list.

Foods to Avoid: While many view potatoes and corn as very healthy additions to the average American diet, don't be fooled. Although both of these foods grow naturally out of the ground, they require both a high level of cultivation (as in settled farming, something our hunter-gatherer ancestors did not do) and a large amount of cooking in order to be fit for consumption.

Potatoes: Similarly to legumes, potatoes contain massive amounts of toxins when raw and can be highly damaging to the human body if consumed in their raw state. While thorough cooking can minimize some of the toxin-load in potatoes, they still retain a certain amount, making them unhealthy for eaters. Potatoes are also a very high carbohydrate food, and although they MUST be cooked in order to be edible, once they are cooked, their carbohydrate content can cause huge sugar spies in the body. Potatoes are a high glycemic index food that can force your body's insulin secretion out of whack and lead your pancreas to be overstressed, leading to fatigue, illness, and inflammation and organ damage. Repeated sugar spikes can lead to type 2 diabetes development as well as obesity and even cognitive decline. For these reasons, potatoes are NOT Paleo.

Corn: Paleo eating is all about making the right, most natural choices for your body and in order to do this, you should ask yourself two questions about any foods you have doubts about. These questions are: "Does this food contain enough nutrition to be eaten?" and "Is this food in anyway toxic?" Our ancestor the Hunter was always looking for prime sources of nutrients that would not pose toxic harm to his body, making survival easier to achieve. If you find that a food is low in nutrition OR that it is highly nutritious but at the same time, that it contains a large toxic load, that food will not help you to survive and thrive and is not an ideal part of your Paleo eating plan.

When it comes to answering those two questions, corn does poorly Corn is neither a good source of human nutrition nor a toxin-free food, making it a bad choice for any diet and especially for a Paleo diet. In the US, we tend to look at corn as a healthy vegetable but this could not be further from the truth. Corn is actually a very harmful grain plant and as we know, grains do not belong on a Paleo eating plan. In fact, corn contains very low levels of nutrients, meaning that although it has some nutrient content, this content is low enough that you would need to eat corn in large amounts to access a useful amount of nutrition. When compared to true Paleo foods like meats, seafood, vegetables, fruits, nuts and seeds, the nutrient value of corn is not high enough to justify its damaging effects.

Corn, like all grains, has a large quantity of prolamins. Prolamins are a type of indigestible protein that can damage your gut as your body tries in vain to break them down. Prolamins lead to leaky gut syndrome and the overgrowth of bad bacteria within your body. Corn is almost completely GMO, making it less of an ancestral, natural food source.

Are Sweet Potatoes Paleo? : This question comes up often because people mistakenly believe that sweet potatoes and potatoes are nearly identical and should be equally non-Paleo. The truth is that many Paleo eaters do well when including sweet potatoes in their diets, in moderation. This is because sweet potatoes and potatoes are actually intrinsically quite different:

Nutrition and Glycemic Index: Many people wrongly point to the caloric and carbohydrate-content similarities between the two types of tubers. For example, 7 ounces of sweet potato provides close to 50 carbs while 7 ounces of normal white potato provides 52 carbs. Very close, you're thinking. In addition, calorically they are also very close with 207 calories for 7 ounces of sweet potato and 221 calories or 7 ounces of normal white potato. If they are so close calorically and carb-wise, then why are sweet potatoes good for you and normal white potatoes not? The answer is that just because the carbs and caloric content of two foods are close, it does not follow that the two foods are equally beneficial. One of the main secrets that make sweet potatoes Paleo-friendly and normal white potatoes a non-Paleo food is in their glycemic loads and glycemic indexes.

- Sweet Potato has a glycemic index **70** of and a glycemic load of **22**

- White Potato has a glycemic index **111** of and a glycemic load of **33**

This means that white potatoes have a glycemic index that is 47 percent higher than the glycemic index of sweet potatoes and that white potatoes' glycemic load is also 44 percent higher than the glycemic load of sweet potatoes. And consider this: Glucose has a glycemic index of 100 and white potatoes have a glycemic index of 111, making them a full 10 percent higher on the glycemic index than PURE SUGAR! What about sweet potatoes Well, their glycemic index is a virtuous 30 percent lower than sugar.

Sweet potatoes are also rich in vitamin A, in comparison to white potatoes. Yet, it is also important to remember that while sweet potatoes are easier on digestion, lower on the glycemic index and glycemic load than white potatoes and more nutrient-dense, they do still have a glycemic index of 70, which is by no means low. Therefore, enjoy sweet potatoes in balanced moderation and do NOT make them a major staple of your Paleo diet, to avoid any risk of developing an insulin resistance problem.

In conclusion, I want to stress that while all Paleo-approved vegetables are a huge boon to your health and fitness they are not to be used improperly. When I say improperly, I mean the way many fad diets have used them over the decades. Vegetables are an addition to your healthy, meat, protein, fat loaded meals and should not become your main foods at all. A lot of people may struggle with this idea because so many low-fat, fad diets have encouraged people (very wrongly!) to replace most of their protein and animal fat calories with vegetables. This is not the Paleo or the ancient, instinctive way of eating that your body requires and if you make vegetables your main meals, you will not succeed in getting the amazing Paleo weight loss, health, energy and mental clarity results that you so richly deserve. Many of the so-called weight loss "experts" who are responsible for the low-fat, high carb diets that have led people into obesity and disease attempt to guilt-trip Paleo eaters into returning to their failed fad diets. Don't lean on those old fad diet habits and don't allow yourself to become scared of not consuming vegetables in excess, because Paleo is not about counting calories, living like a rabbit or starving yourself. Instead, it is all about nourishing your body so that it naturally and willingly loosens its grip on those stubborn pounds and allows you to access great health, energy, mood and mental sharpness at the same time!

Chapter 7:
Paleo and Legumes: Why Legumes are Not Paleo and Not as Good For You as You Thought!

We've heard it over and over, a million times from those high school nutrition classes all the way to the doctor's office and even in some top health and fitness magazines: "Eat your legumes, they are some of the healthiest foods you'll ever come across!"

So legumes must be Paleo, right? Well, actually, they're not. I know that this may come as a huge surprise to many people who've always been led to believe that legumes were an intrinsic, necessary and major part of a healthy weight-loss diet, but the truth is, legumes would have been virtually unrecognizable and foreign to our ancestor, the Hunter and they would definitely not have been consumed by him for energy, health or strength. Why, you may wonder? The answer is very simple: Legumes are NOT a true, ancestral Paleo food.

To get a clearer understanding of what makes legumes completely unsuitable for a truly Paleo way of eating plan, lets first take a look at which items fall under the classification of legumes:

Non-Paleo Legumes:

- Lentils

- Beans

- Peas

- Peanuts

- Soy Beans

- Small White Beans

- Red Beans

- Pinto Beans

- Mexican Black Beans

- Mexican Red Bean

- Mung Beans

- Split Peas

- Boston Beans

- Chickpeas

- Chili Beans

- Fava Beans

- Field Peas

- And All Other Types of Beans, Peas and Peanuts

While legumes manage to avoid the extremely negative reputation the grains do, they are still on the "eliminate "list. When it comes to achieving truly amazing paleo results, don't let legumes stand in your way!

The Truth About Legumes: We tend to hear about how healthy and jam-packed with nutrients legumes are and in one sense, that is true. When legumes are in their raw state, they do contain quite a large amount of important nutrients. However, the problem with legumes arises when they are cooked. Cooked legumes lose the vast majority of their useful nutrients and are no longer much use to our bodies, making their rich nutrition content largely a myth.

Legumes Can Block Nutrients: While legumes do have a moderate amount of such vital nutrients as magnesium, calcium, potassium and iron, these nutrients are not able to last beyond the consumption process. Once legumes are ingested, these nutrients are not taken in by the body.

Legumes Have High Phytate Content: Legumes have got yet another problem to pose to our bodies. They are plagued with very large doses of phytates. Phytates are naturally occurring components found in almost every type of legume. These phytates do not allow the minerals that you eat to be absorbed into your body properly. Phytates can block the absorption and utilization of nutrients to the point that many unaware consumers of legumes may actually find that they develop iron deficiencies and anemia, from long term legume eating. Phytates also have the unfortunate tendency to prevent the necessary digestive enzymes amylase and pepsin from doing their digestive work. This results in a longer, more difficult digestive process and can lead to inflammation bloating and fatigue.

Legumes Are Loaded with Lectins: As if the lack of nutrients after cooking, difficult digestion and phytate content weren't enough to make legumes a distinctly unhealthy and non-Paleo food, legumes are also loaded with large quantities of tough to handle anti-nutrients called lectins! Numerous studies have shown that regular exposure to these lectins can end up leading to a severely inflamed gut and that this inflammation can in turn, even lead to increased permeability of the intestinal lining otherwise known as "leaky gut syndrome". When leaky gut syndrome persists, it can often end up leading to a failure of your body's ability to absorb or utilize many different vitamins and minerals. In the long term leaky gut syndrome can also result in the development of serious food allergies as your body produces harsh antibodies in order to launch a counterattack against these foreign invader-like lectins. What ends up occurring is that your body's immune system ends up mistakenly launching these antibodies against your own tissue. This kind of low-grade long term inflammation often also leads to such manifestations as rheumatoid arthritis and other autoimmune disorders, as well as an inflamed brain.

You should definitely steer clear of legumes in order to protect yourself , if you have any pre-existing autoimmune conditions or high inflammation markers, because consuming legumes can make your problem much worse!

Legumes Are Packed with Protease Inhibitors: Legumes are also filled with inhibitors that disrupt and halt the work of protease in your body. Protease is an enzyme that your body naturally releases in order to effectively break down proteins for digestion. However, the protease inhibitors inherent in all legumes prevent this important function and the results range from food allergies to long term inflammation and a permeable leaky gut. Not only are these symptoms painful but they also can be the first signs of a serious protein deficiency. The simple fact is that, when you regularly consume legumes, no matter how many high-quality proteins you include in your diet, your body will be severely protein deficient because of the protease inhibitors found in these legumes.

Legumes Contain Saponins and FODMAPS: Legumes also contain very high amounts of saponins. Saponins can wreak serious destruction within your intestines by binding themselves to the cells of the intestines and then slipping into your blood, carrying with them many harmful toxins, chemicals and bacteria. Long term consumption of legumes can lead to saponin-led red blood cell membrane damage.

Legumes also present another hazard in the form of FODMAPS, carbohydrates that a large portion of people find hard to digest. Galectin and other FODMAPS present in legumes can cause unpleasant side effects ranging from headaches, rashes, excessive gas production and lethargy to ADHD, impaired cognitive abilities and anxiety.

Legumes and Phytoestrogens: High levels of phytoestrogens found within legumes can present a wide and severe array of problems. Because phytoestrogens are similar enough to true estrogen to be able to mimic its effects within your body, they can turn on your estrogen receptors. They put out signals that can stimulate too much estrogen production, which can completely upset the delicate hormonal balance within your body. This imbalance can the lead to the emergence of asthma and other breathing difficulties, fertility problems, various cancers (particularly ovarian, uterine, bladder and breast cancers) and even up your risk of having Alzheimer's and other types of cognitive disorders. The BPA found in the linings of many canned legume products can also disrupt hormonal functions and create imbalances that lead to development issues, fertility problems, breast and prostate cancers as well as an increased risk of cardiovascular disease and even diabetes development.

A Last Word on Legumes: For all of the reasons above and more, legumes are not considered a health part of any Paleo eating plan. However, many vegetarians and those who consume lower amounts of animal protein may find that only legumes provide them with sufficient plant doses. Still, this protein content is not a reason for Paleo eaters to consider adding legumes to their diet because their protein content, while high for a plant, is nothing special when compared to protein-rich animal sources and as we discussed, due to legumes' protease inhibitors, much of their protein is not bioavailable to humans anyway! Legumes also add unnecessary amounts of carbohydrates to your meal plan without providing enough nutritional content to warrant this increase and as we all know, too many carbohydrates can slow down your weight loss and spike your blood sugar levels (not to mention contribute to certain conditions such as candida within the body, making autoimmune disorders worse). With all of the potential pitfalls and not enough benefits to offer, I advise that you do with legumes what our wise ancestor the Hunter did- ignore them completely!

Chapter 8:
The Big Fat Secret: Fat Makes You Fitter, NOT Fatter!

Picture this: It's several millennia ago and after a long hard day of careful stalking, the Hunter has just scored his prey, a large fine specimen of big game. He now crouches over his catch with his family, enjoying the taste of fresh meat. Do you think that the Hunter and his family only eat the leaner cuts of meat from the animal he's just killed? Do you imagine them throwing everything else away as "unhealthy"? Of course not! When it came to meat, our early ancestors (and many remaining hunter-gatherer tribes today) always preferred the richest sources of nutrition such as dark organ meats, bone marrow and yes, lots and lots of fresh, good-for-you animal fats!

Fast forward to the present and what do you see at the typical American dinner table? Modern man and his family are busily trimming off the best, most fatty parts of their already lean steaks. They are careful to only use non-fat spreads instead of butter and they would never, ever even consider eating full fat anything! Why? Because modern man is constantly warned by his doctor, nutritionist, the media and even the "official" food pyramid that fat equals bad. That's why we see so many people removing the rich fat from their protein sources before cooking, essentially taking something highly nutritious and absolutely VITAL to good health, and just tossing it into the trash! If the Hunter could see how we disregard the best parts of the animal, he wouldn't be able to believe his eyes! We have been told that fat is public enemy number one, the biggest threat to our health and our waistlines, so many times that even though no real proof has ever been provided to backup these claims, we have been conditioned to simply accept them as true. Although our minds may be swayed by those low-fat messages, our bodies, however, are not so easy to fool. In the past few decades, when the widespread villainization of saturated fat began to reach fever pitch, we ,as a society, completely turned our backs on millennia of ancient and healthful eating wisdom that our species had always practiced, instead opting for reduced fat, low fat, no fat everything. We trimmed, skimmed, scraped and separated the valuable fat out of all of our food items, until we were left with a diet full of dry, tasteless, bulky grains, promoted as the most beneficial way of eating for well-being, weight loss and longevity.

And what did our bodies do? To the shock and horror of all those anti-fat, whole grain doctors and experts, the more we cut fat out of our lives, the more fat our bodies stubbornly held on to. The more we allowed food manufacturers to literally suck the fat out of our meals, the less fit, healthy and slim we became. In fact, as you read this today, at the height of the no fat hysteria, we as humans have become more physically fat, heavy and unfit as a species, than we have ever been at any other time in our collective human history! So how does that add up? If eating fat makes you fat, then why did reducing or even completely removing fat from our diets result in dramatic, rapid and massive weight gain? To really understand what happened to our bodies during the recent (and still on-going) no fat revolution and to learn how to undo the damage, you have to forget everything you've been told in health class, on TV, by diet books and doctors alike. Because the simple fact is, we now unanimously know that the no fat movement was totally wrong: It's a **lack** of fat that makes humans fatter and in fact, the higher our consumption of saturated fats, the leaner, fitter, slimmer, healthier, smarter and even happier we become! Of course, the "low fat, no fat gurus" haven't been very thrilled about this new shift in thinking, but although they try to hold it back with their half-baked, groundless theories, the full fat Paleo train has left the station and millions of healthier, lighter and more satisfied people are onboard! When it comes to going Paleo, although other health changes in the diet are just as important to make, no other change leads to the amazing, almost unbelievable physical, mental and even emotional results that switching into full fat mode brings. If you're looking to totally transform the way you look, feel and perform mentally and physically, the full saturated fat Paleo movement is EXACTLY what you need!

Affordable, Delicious & Nutritious: Saturated Fat is the Perfect Body, Brain and Budget-Friendly Food! Not only is fat a fantastic, delicious and highly nutrient rich healthy item to add to your diet, I want you to know that it is also perhaps the least expensive Paleo item out there. That's right, adding fat to your diet will shrink your grocery bill AND your waist line! That's because, with all of the mass anti-fat hysteria circulating in the media and the world of conventional medicine today, what was once the most highly prized food item for health and well-being has become universally feared. Grocery stores know they can get away with charging you an arm and a leg for supposedly "healthy" and "weight loss promoting" foods like lean meat and chicken breast, while the real health food star fat has been given such an undeserved bad reputation that you can buy as much of it as you want for a very low price.

 And that's great news for those of us who don't want our Paleo diet to break the bank. When you choose fattier cuts of meat or higher fat content ground beef, you'll see that not only do the pounds drop right off of you and the aches, pains and fatigue you've struggled with disappear, but the strain on your wallet from buying those unnecessarily expensive, less healthy lean meats will also vanish. What's not to love about fat? It makes you skinny, sharper, stronger, happier and works better, faster and more cheaply than any costly supplement or diet food out there! Are you ready to start eating the way your body was designed to eat, never fell hungry or unsatisfied again and lose some serious weight to boot?

Did you know that fats make up a portion of each and every cell in your body? Let's take a look at some of the incredible science solidly supporting an increased consumption of saturated fat for better health: (You may need these facts to argue against the baseless "anti-fat" campaigners in your own life, when they see you reaching for the real butter!)

Fat Myth # 1: Eating Fat Will Make You Get Fat: This theory sounds like it should make sense but in all truth, it simply doesn't. Our ancient ancestor, the Hunter, was lean, strong and had a much higher proportion of muscle than fat in his body. Yet, he ate as much pure animal fat as he could possibly get his hands on. What about the average human being today? The sad fact is that our no fat diets have not done us any favors, leaving us overweight or obese, tired, with little or no muscle mass and with huge, hard to lose stores of unwanted fat. Fat is, in reality, the best weight loss food possible. It works in several powerful ways:

- When you replace your high carbohydrate diet with a diet rich in saturated fat, your body's inulin production and release process is totally transformed. In order to manage sugar, insulin is released in large amounts when you consume carbohydrates but when you replace these carbs with fats, you achieve a much lower level of insulin and you are able to access fat as the primary fuel for your body.

- Biologically, eating lots of saturated fat makes your body very efficient at burning fat whereas low fat diets are bad for adipokines, hormones that are in charge of fat-burning. When you eat enough fat, adipokines are able to ramp up your metabolism and even decrease your appetite.

- If you've ever eaten a largely carb-loaded diet, you know that it is always accompanied by pesky hunger pangs and cravings that make overeating inevitable. That's not the case when it comes to fat. Because saturated fats cause the release of appetite regulating hormones CCK and PYY, eating a Paleo diet full of rich, satisfying fats leaves you always feeling satiated and never in danger of gorging on unhealthy foods.

Fat Myth #2: Eating Saturated Fat Will Give You Cancer: This is an often repeated myth that has never been properly backed up with solid research, but the scare tactics used in making such a claim have been enough to keep most people away from fat, in the mistaken belief that they could be upping their own cancer risk. So what do the facts say? Just the opposite of this, actually: A series of scientific studies carried out on the consumption of super-saturated fat beef tallow found that not only does eating saturated animal fat NOT cause cancer, it can actually improve the cancer-fighting and preventative power of CLA (Conjugated Linoleic Acid)! In one study, eating beef tallow even clearly led to the ability to fend off mammary tumor development! There is one VERY important thing to note, however: If you want to replicate these results in your own life, make sure that the beef tallow you are eating is from pastured, not commercially grain-fed cows. This is absolutely essential because the fat of grass-fed, pastured cows contains much larger amounts of naturally conjugated linoleic acid than the fat from grain-fed, commercially raised cows, making pastured beef tallow a super anti-carcinogenic food!

Fat Myth # 3: Eating Saturated Fat Is Bad for Your Cholesterol Levels and Your Overall Cardiovascular Health: This may be the most cited concern when people first hear about making the switch to more fat consumption. But the truth is that this concern is unfounded and based on outdated studies that do not prove the point. In fact, the studies meant to prove cholesterol is formed from saturated fat consumption were carried out on rabbits! Rabbits were force fed huge amounts of saturated fats and of course became quite ill. This was used to postulate that saturated fat can kill us. But as we know, humans are NOT rabbits. Rabbits are herbivores that never naturally eat sources of saturated fats so it makes sense that large amounts of saturated fat would sicken them. We, however, have always used and even preferred saturated fats as a source of nutrition and it does not harm us in the same way. Our hearts and indeed our cholesterol levels need plenty of good, saturated fats for health and proper balance. In fact, studies carried out on humans(as opposed to rabbits) show us that consuming a diet high in saturated fat can even lower levels of the bad cholesterol LDL and change the nature of the LDL particles themselves from the highly harmful dense small hard particles that cause heart attacks into the large fluffy and harmless kind. Eating plentiful amounts of fat also increases the amount of good HDL cholesterol in our bodies, making us more resistant to heart disease.

Fat Myth # 4: Eating Saturated Fat Will Generally Make You Sicker: Again, this statement is also completely unfounded. On the other hand, there is plenty of evidence that the reverse is true. Adding saturated fat to your diet can actually improve your health across the board. Let's check out the evidence:

- A good amount of dietary saturated fat protects the liver from disease by allowing it to properly flush out toxins and excess fatty accumulation.

- A diet of saturated fat is lung protective: Our lungs have air spaces within them and these air spaces are covered with a substance that is made up of only fat. When we eat enough saturated fat, these spaces and our lungs in general are healthy. When we fail to get enough saturated fat in our diets, these air spaces actually fail, causing a collapse and leading to lung diseases and disorders. In fact, the recent rise of asthma in our population may be linked to the rise of the low and no fat "health" craze. Think about it, a lack of fat can make it hard to do the one thing we can't survive without: breathe!

- Fat soluble vitamins such as vitamin A, vitamin D, vitamin E and vitamin K are found in plenty within saturated fat sources like butter and beef tallow. This makes these fatty foods a complete nutrient package because these vitamins will not be properly absorbed without fat, but when you eat the saturated fats that contain these vitamins, you are giving your body the most bioavailable, soluble and active versions of these vitamins.

- Saturated fats often contain anti-microbe properties, making them a necessary tool to fend off common microbial-led diseases and infections. When you want to ward off common infections and keep your immune system healthy, make sure you stock up on some good protective saturated fats.

Fat Myth # 5: Fat Is Bad for Your Brain: Now this myth is particularly ridiculous and is often used by vegans and vegetarians to explain their belief that fat is not necessary for intelligence. Well, that may be true when it comes to naturally vegetarian animals like rabbits but it certainly does NOT hold true for most mammals and most especially not for human beings. Our brains absolutely need saturated fat and they need it in large amounts. The brains of human beings are made up of almost 60 % fat content. This fat content is composed of essential fatty acids like Omega 3s that are vital for the full and proper development of the human brain. In addition, fat makes up the myelin sheath that covers neurons, making them very important in the nerve, neuron signaling process. When you look at it like that, a low or no fat diet is the fastest way to harm your brain and reduce your intelligence ever. And that's not just a theory! Studies have shown that vegetarians who completely eschew saturated fats lose up to 5% of their brain mass in only 5 years! What happens to paleo saturated fat eaters is the exact opposite: Instead of losing precious brain mass, we lose unwanted pounds off of our waists and bodies while improving our brains' capabilities and health!

Fat Myth # 6: OK, Eating Fat May Make You Skinny, Healthy and Smart but...You'll be Really, Really Tired: Nice try, but wrong again. This is the myth that many nutritionists fall back on once you've disproved all of the tired theories about heart health and brain power to them. You see, for a very long time, we were taught that carbohydrate consumption was the best possible way we could obtain food energy and stay active. Is this true? A simple way to debunk this myth is by eating a big whole wheat bagel with a low fat non-butter spread. After about an hour, you feel like passing out from exhaustion, right? That's because carbs are only short term sugar rush sources, NOT real energy sources. Now, see how you feel after a Paleo saturated fat meal such as bacon, eggs and butter. You'll find that not only are you not passing out with fatigue, you are actually more energetic, clear-headed, alert and awake than ever. This is because fats provide you with a nice, clean burning, and long-lasting source of energy. And did you know that when it comes to energy amount, fats have carbs beat by a long way? Yes, fat is actually our main source of stored energy and offers us 3 times the amount of energy that carbohydrates can provide. Your body can break down and utilize triglycerides for energy and your brains neurons use it as a go to source of energy in times of stress and duress. Unlike carbohydrates, one meal of fat can fuel us for many hours while carbohydrates must be frequently and continually consumed throughout the day to avoid a slump.

As we've seen, far from being the much maligned substance that we've been told to fear, fat is actually a powerful tool for human well-being. In fact, nothing works to help you drop those pounds and improve your overall health like saturated fats. Now that we've debunked the most common anti-fat myths, join me in the next chapter to get all the information you need to use fat in the most effective way possible and turn your body into a lean, mean, fat-burning machine!

Chapter 9:
Utilizing Fats the Paleo Way

Now that you've gone beyond the first few weeks of the Paleo of eating, you've probably seen massive changes in your energy and even your body. However, when it comes to getting the most incredible results that this way of eating has to offer, it's all about the fats. If you're at this point, you're now ready to learn the tips and techniques that make fats your best friend.

Let's get to it!

Are All Fats Equal?

The answer to that is a definite no. When I mention the amazing health benefits of fat, I'm not talking about just any old fat. The fact is, trans fats that are found in most commercially prepared goods, from snacks and sauces to desserts and even salad dressings, will do you so much harm that they absolutely do not belong on your Paleo eating plan. Fats found in highly processed cold cuts won't do you much good either, as they are the type most likely to form Advanced Glycation End Products (AGEs), substances that basically destroy your DNA and bring you to the brink of rapid ageing. Within the broad field of fats, there are many, many wonderful truly Paleo fats that were just as likely to be enjoyed by the Hunter as by modern man and which are loaded with exactly the health-helping properties that the human body has always and will always need. There are also a few fats that MUST be avoided, and that's what this chapter is all about: Sorting out the good from the bad and helping you to use the right fats in the best, most beneficial, most healthy and most affordable way for Paleo results that'll have you over the moon with joy but won't end up costing you the Earth.

An Easy Guide to Paleo Fats:

How to tell a Healthy fat from an unhealthy fat:

- Healthy fats tend to be made up of a higher percentage of saturated fatty acids as opposed to unsaturated fatty acids

- Healthy fats tend to be more stable

- Healthy animal fats usually come from pastured, grass-fed animals

- Healthy plant fats usually come from organic and/or untampered -with plant sources

Unhealthy Fats:

- Unhealthy fats tend to be made up of more unsaturated fatty acids than saturated fatty acids

- Unhealthy fats are less stable

- Unhealthy animal fats come from grain-fed, heavily medicated (with antibiotics), caged in and improperly commercially raised animals

- Unhealthy plant fats tend to come from pesticide laden, chemically processed sources

Paleo Fats to Love:

1. **Coconut:** Who would have ever believed that one of your body's fattest and best friends actually grows on trees? Well, it's true and while the Paleo diet is often heavily skewed towards things that moo, grunt and move, in this case, it's a plant that's taking top honors. Coconut is loaded with ultra-beneficial saturated fat but unlike other sources of saturated fat, over 50 % of coconut's fat content is made up of lauric acid. Lauric acid is an important lipid that boasts a wide range

of amazing properties from being a major cholesterol profile helper to even thwarting the efforts of bad bacteria as well as anti-abdominal visceral fat effects. So if you're looking for a way to get washboard abs, low cholesterol levels and stay protected from all manner of harmful infectious diseases at the same time, Paleo's star food, coconut fat is your best bet! In fact, a study in which participants were dosed with daily spoonfuls of coconut oil saw the subjects' waist sizes shrink rapidly! You can use coconut fat (coconut fat is an oil that actually comes in a solid form, at room temperature) to cook, bake, roast and even fry anything from meats to veggies and even sweeter Paleo treats. Additionally, Paleo people love to dose their morning coffee with a dollop of this delicately scented and tasty oil to turn their morning hot drink into a weight loss weapon that keeps them svelte and leaves them feeling energetic for hours! Try it for a taste you'll love and weight loss results you won't believe!

2. **Beef Tallow:** The most budget-friendly, nutrient rich fat of all! Even grass-fed beef tallow is super cheap (and often even free!) because all of the anti-fat hype has

wrongly forced it off the menus of most people! You can easily score a large amount of valuable, grass-fed beef tallow for a mere pittance from your local grass-fed beef purveyor or farm. Often, if you are buying meat from them, they'll be more than happy to throw in the beef tallow for free! But just because beef tallow is highly affordable does not mean it skimps on the benefits at ALL. Grass-fed beef tallow is chockfull of the extremely effective fat- burning, muscle mass increasing fatty acid Conjugated Linoleic Acid (CLA). Even the low-fat crowd can't resist the benefits of CLA so they try to buy it in pill form in vitamin and supplement stores for insanely high prices, but guess what? The CLA in those stores comes mainly from safflower oil, a very poor source indeed. When you add the dirt-cheap but super-nutritious grass-fed beef tallow you got from your local farm or meat source to your diet, you're getting a whopping 300 to 500 times the potent CLA power that can be found in any other source!

Here's a quick rundown of some of the benefits of the CLA found in beef tallow:

Studies prove that CLA is ant-cancerous, both preventing and thwarting the emergence and growth of malignant tumors in the body. Studies also show that CLA is just as powerful when it comes to dousing the flames of inflammation as it is when it comes to burning fat! And CLA can help to quell painful inflammatory conditions like Crohn's disease, with regular consumption. So how do you get in on all of these beef tallow benefits? Well, here's a simple guide:

Obtaining the Source:

Heading over to your local farmers' market is a great way to access some prime beef fat for tallow rendering. If there's a beef provider there with good grass-fed practices they will probably be glad to give you the fat you need to get beef tallow from at rock bottom prices or even, for free!

OK, so no you've got a whole hunk of beef fat. What's next? You simply trim any excess meat off the fat (save the meat for addition to your supply of grass-fed meat based meals!) and then cut the fat into very small pieces. Place these pieces into a stainless steel pot and make sure that the fat only comes to about half way up the pot. Next, place on the stove at a medium- to low temperature and stir every so often to ensure that nothing is burning and that the fat is being evenly cooked.

The pieces of fat should begin to really melt down after about half an hour of simmering. Now that you've got this golden yellow liquid in the pot, you can ladle it into very clean glass containers and cover with a good, airtight lid.

Storage: You can store the rendered down beef tallow in the refrigerator or in a cool, dark cabinet or panty, where it won't be disturbed by the sun's rays or excessive heat. The liquid will solidify into a pale creamy colored solid, butter-like concoction when it cools to room temperature. To use, simply stick in a clean spoon and remove a chunk for cooking.

Now, you've got an incredible-tasting cooking fat to add to everything from stews and baked vegetables to your morning eggs and the best part is, this affordable and amazing fat will help you to naturally burn body fat and fend off disease, all day long!

3. **Full Fat, Real, Raw Butter:** Long gone are the days when we could be led to believe that butter is unequivocally evil. With its rich nutrient-packed creamy deliciousness, butter made from grass-fed raw milk sources is BACK on our menus in a big way! If you're new to Paleo, you probably bought margarine or some other low-fat artificial butter-like spread instead of getting the real thing in the past, because conventional health food experts have been mistakenly claiming that butter leads to a whole host of diseases. But Paleo is completely different. While it's true that our ancestor the Hunter wasn't out there milking wild wildebeests for milk and making butter from it, butter and other full fat raw dairy may still be the most Paleo food items around in terms of sheer nutrition and fat content! If you're still using margarine on your food, read these benefits of butter and stop now. You'll be saving yourself from numerous illnesses, obesity and fatigue, as well as improving your mental abilities and emotional stability.

Butter simply beats margarine on every level. For one thing, butter is real. It comes from a natural source not a laboratory. It is simply, almost instinctively produced. Unlike margarine, it is not the result of a long, complicated and very unhealthy commercial process that turns dry corn into a "creamy" spread. "But", you may exclaim, "Margarine is heart-healthy. It says so right there on the package." Well, the heart-healthy label comes from margarine's total lack of natural, good saturated fats. Because margarine is severely lacking fat, doctors and nutritionists have promoted it as the best spread for your heart for decades. But the truth of the matter is that this lack of fat can actually lead to a buildup of hard dense LDL particles in your arteries, the kind that lead to heart attacks! Butter, on the other hand, turns your cholesterol into soft, harmless, fluffy particles that do no damage, while at the same time upping your levels of good HDL cholesterol. In all reality, real butter (and not fake margarine) should be the one that is labelled heart-healthy!

Margarine and other low-fat spreads are made of trans fats. This alone is enough to make them the absolute worst thing you could do to your heart and your whole body and brain. Trans fats make your bad LDL cholesterol levels skyrocket while making your good HDL cholesterol levels plummet. In addition, studies have shown that there is a definite link between trans fats consumption and the development of type 2 diabetes, major obesity, arterial blocks, strokes and even autoimmune disorders! So, we know that margarine definitely does not belong anywhere near your new Paleo lifestyle. Now, let's take a look at the reasons why butter rules the roost, when it comes to health:

Butter is intensely nutrient rich. Loaded with plenty of fat-soluble vitamins such as vitamin A, vitamin D, vitamin E and vitamin K, butter can help with everything from the healthy functioning of the endocrine system to the protection of the eyes. Its vitamin D content is especially important as vitamin D is hard to obtain but is necessary to ward off autoimmune disorders, weight loss, depression and even mental illness. Vitamin D has also been shown to fight cancer, so get a nice, large dollop of raw milk butter and enjoy the rewards.

Butter is also just as rich in minerals. Important trace minerals like zinc, copper, chromium and manganese are all present inside butter's creamy goodness. Want a major does of the antioxidant powerhouse selenium? A helping of butter will provide you with more of this vital nutrient than you can find in the fish herring! Butter is also an excellently balanced source of omega 3 fatty acids, because its omega 3 to omega 6 ratio is correct. It's also rich in plenteous amounts of short-chain and medium-chain fatty acids, making it essential for your immune system's functions and can help to make weight loss easy and natural. Abundant amounts of Conjugated Linoleic Acid make their appearance in butter as well, leaving you with anti-cancer, anti-weight gain and anti-inflammatory benefits. Humans have always used fatty foods to combat stiffness, dryness and irritation and butter is particularly useful in this area as well. It contains a substance that is similar to hormones called the Wulzen factor which fights off arthritis and other types of inflammation and stiffness in the joints.

Budget Smart Move: Although many types of foods can be switched out for others, when it comes to butter, it is best to always make sure that you are consuming the raw, grass-fed kind. As you need relatively smaller amounts to boost your good fat intake, you can easily add this to your diet without too much price strain. However, always remember that many small scale local dairy farmers would only be too happy to cut a favorable deal with you, if you are interested in buying fresh, raw butter straight from the source. Look for such farmers online or visit a farmers' market to get information.

Chapter 10:
How the Wrong Cooking Oils Could Secretly Be Making You Sicker, Fatter and Sadder!

Did you know that Omega-6 fats only made up less than 3 percent of all daily calories consumed, only 100 years ago? And what about their presence in the average American diet today? That number has gone up to 10 percent of all daily calories and along with the rise of omega-6 in our diets, both rates of bipolar disorders and cardiovascular-related deaths have shot up! Are these merely coincidences or linked occurrences?

Both omega-6 and omega-3 fats have important functions in the body. Once these fats are consumed they are transformed into eicosanoids in your body. Eicosanoids are used to relay messages within your body, signaling it to launch inflammatory or immune reactions. One type of eicosanoids, called an endocannabinoid, is even in charge of regulating the human appetite, mood and memory. When in proper balance, omega-6 fats and omega-3 fats are capable of providing your body with very important functions. However, when that balance is upset, serious havoc breaks loose!

These days, the average American gets far more omega-6 fats than omega-3 fats, setting the stage for severe harm. This is because getting the majority of your eicosanoids and endocannabinoids from omega-6 sources rather than omega-3 sources can leave your appetite out of control, making your ravenous and stopping your from being satisfied with your meals. This state also causes extreme mood swings and can even lead to major illnesses and deaths. This is due to the fact that while omega-3 fats are intensely anti-inflammatory omega-6 fats are just the opposite in large amounts, causing chronic, high levels of inflammation and leading to the development of many types of cancers, emotional and mental disturbances, depression and even heart disease! This may seem like quite a startling list of effects and it is even more disturbing when you realize that all of this damage is coming from one major source: Cooking oil!

Due to an abundance of omega-6 loaded cooking oils, many Americans are raising their risk of developing many terrifying mental and physical disorders that destroy their quality of life AND can cause premature death.

How YOU Can Put A Stop to the Omega-6 Madness:

Most people, even on a Paleo diet, look very carefully at the meats, fruits, vegetables, nuts and seeds they consume but unfortunately, they do not pay the same amount of attention to the oils they cook with. This problem is compounded further by the fact that many of the worst omega-6 offending oils are labelled "heart-healthy" , "all-natural" and other misleading labels, causing the average consumer to believe they are making an excellent health choice by selecting and using these oils.

That's why I want you to be forearmed with these very important but super-simple tips that can help save you from madness, illness, weight gain and other unpleasant side effects of the omega-6 imbalance:

1. Start by selecting low omega-6 cooking oil: The very best cooking oils you can use are ultra-high in good saturated fats and ultra-low in omega-6 fats. Not only do omega-6 fats cause an eicosanoid and endocannabinoids the serious problems outlined above, they are also very far from being stable. Omega-6 fats quickly go bad, turning rancid in the cooking and storing

process and they may even be rancid while sitting in the aisle s of your grocery store! Not only are rancid oils highly unpleasant to the taste, they are also unsuitable for the human body to utilize. This often leads to the diseases-causing systemic inflammation that omega-6 oils cause.

2. Look for very low omega-6 content oil with a low smoke point: The smoke point basically means the point during cooking that an oil begins to breakdown and smoke .This point could also be called the "flavor and health benefits-loss point" because that's exactly what happens when these oils reach their smoke point. Chose a good, stable, oil low in omega-6 fats for fantastic flavor and safe nutrition.

3. Always Choose a Less Processed Oil: All oils undergo a certain amount of processing but do your best to choose one with minimal processing. This means that you'd do well to go for oil from an "oily" source. Seed and vegetable oils are harmful because they must be heavily processed in order to produce oils from seeds and vegetables, which are not naturally "oily". Olive oil on the other

hand, comes from a source rich in natural oils and requires almost no processing to collect that oil. Seeds and vegetables are processed with the dangerous carcinogen hexane, in order to produce oil from them. Because these oils are not naturally occurring, huge amounts of preservatives are also added into them to obtain a longer shelf life!

4. **Don't Be Fooled by Smoke:** Many processed vegetable and seed oils have much higher smoke points than healthy, minimally processed oils like olive oil and coconut oil. However, just because there's smoke doesn't mean there's fire. In other words, natural oils may smoke more quickly but they still do not cause the inflammation and disease that these artificial processed oils do. Always go for low omega-6 oils from naturally oil-producing sources first and worry about smoke point last.

5. **Remember that Most Seed Oils and Vegetable Oils are GMO:** We can't be sure about the impact this may have on human health but if you are trying to eat as naturally and as ancestrally as possible, remember that your hunter-gatherer

ancestors were not trying to squeeze oil out of seeds and vegetables! This applies directly to all seed oils and particularly to canola, corn and soy oils!

Avoid These Oils At All Times:

Corn Oil: Mostly Omega-6, highly unstable and loaded with chemicals

Canola Oil: Also mostly omega-6, packed with trans-fats, unstable and also full of chemicals

Safflower Oil: labelled "healthy" but in reality a terrible oil. Safflower oil is lacking in any stability and is highly inflammatory as well as requiring harsh chemical processing to produce a drop of oil.

Soybean Oil: Often called GMO juice, soybean oil is packed with unstable, polyunsaturated fats and its omega-6 content makes it an inflammation fire starter.

All Seed Oils: Sunflower Seed, Grape Seed, Cottonseed, and Flax Seed Oils: When you get your oil from seeds, you basically get a very skewed omega-6 to omega-3 ratio. These oils are also not ideal for cooking.

Good Oils to Use in Moderation:

Walnut oil (still higher in omega-6, so use only rarely)

Sesame oil (still higher in omega-6, so use only rarely)

The Best Oils to Use in Abundance:

Ghee

Extra-Virgin Olive Oil (Does have a lower smoke point so use only for light, low-heat cooking. It is excellent for cold dishes, however)

Coconut Oil

Grass-fed Raw Milk Butter

Pure Unadulterated Lard

Grass-fed Beef Tallow (Very affordable!)

Duck Fat

Making this very simple switch from unbalanced, unstable and unhealthy omea-6 oils to natural, unprocessed and saturated fat-rich oils may be the move that will fix any underlying health issues or inflammation that you have been battling. Try this fantastically easy Paleo step and watch the rewards roll in!

Chapter 11:
Paleo Beverages Part 1: What's In, What's Out and How to Decide

The original role model of the Paleo diet, the Hunter, was a man of relatively simple tastes and means. Compared to the thousands of beverage types and options we have in supermarkets and vending machines today, the Hunter's drink selections definitely look meager. So what can you drink on a Paleo diet and lifestyle plan? Well, depending on the rules provided by different experts, the answer varies. Some Paleo plans insist that hunter-gatherer's only had access to water and that modern man should emulate their lifestyle to the letter. But that would mean having to ignore a lot of anecdotal, traditional and scientific date proving that certain beverages that may not have been easily available to the Hunter are highly beneficial to your body and should be included in your diet. The advice I'm going to give you regarding beverage choices is based on the entire philosophy of this book. Paleo is not a gimmicky, "lose weight quick, put it back on even quicker" type of diet. It's a long-term even life-long way of being that provides untold healing and nourishment to your body and brain. That's why it is so important that you feel you can stick with it. Most diets are either ridiculously lenient (to the point where everything is allowed, and they just don't work) while other diets are so regulated, rigid and unnecessarily inflexible that they are like walking on a tightrope. You may be able to take a few unsteady steps but sooner rather than later, you're bound to fall off. The Paleo diet is all about sustainability, helping you to stay on the most beneficial eating, exercise and lifestyle habits path for as long as possible. This is why, when you go Paleo, you find that you don't ever want to look back, let alone GO back to those painful, expensive and unhelpful diet failures in the past.

So when it comes to choosing beverages, (as with almost every facet of the Paleo diet) I say, make the Hunter your target but don't feel that you have to hit the bull's eye every single time. The single most important factor in deciding what to eat, drink, or do on a diet plan is the way that the option in question makes you feel. With that being said, let's take a look at how various drinks stack up on the Paleo diet:

Water: Drink as much water as possible. Pure, clean water is perhaps the most Paleo thing you can put into your body. The Hunter was constantly on the lookout for fresh sources of this valuable and vital substance and today, your body needs it just as much. The human body is more than 50% water and the benefits that this original quencher provides to you ranges from improved digestion and detoxification to clear glowing skin, higher energy, better mental clarity and healthier organs! So let's talk amounts. Every dietician will tell you that you need at least 8 glasses of water a day. But did the Hunter have access to that much drinking water? Depending on the time of year and the weather conditions (i.e. drought versus rain fall) the Hunter probably did not enjoy year-round access to that much clean drinking water. However, that's not to say that if he did suddenly find a huge supply of water, he wouldn't have made full use of it. The simple fact is that being thirsty is not the first sign of dehydration. Your body is constantly losing precious moisture throughout the day and even while sleeping. When you look at the list of ways your body needs water above, you quickly realize that limiting your intake below 8 glasses is not a great idea. So what's the Paleo recommendation? Drink water regularly. Make sure it your number 1 beverage of choice. Don't waste your money on insanely wasteful packs of bottled water. The plastic in the bottles will seep hormone disrupting substances into your water and body. Additionally, these plastic bottles are often left in the sun, compounding the chemical leaching problem even further. It is also important to note that "Pure Spring Water" the water in most fancy bottled water actually comes from a tap water source in the first place! Save both your money and your health by opting for non-bottled water. Instead , install a good filtration system on your tap water source to remove the more harmful elements that exist in water thanks to modern day living and pour your daily supply of drinking water into a non-plastic container. This way, you'll have clean, fresh water available to you all day while avoiding both the risk of chemical contamination and the unnecessary expense of shelling out for unhealthy and wasteful bottled water!

Forget all of those super-pricey "healthy" waters like waters with vitamins and minerals added in during the production process, too. These vitamin waters are not only lacking in any real benefit, they are also often loaded with sugar, artificial sweeteners and neon food coloring that will directly damage your body and brain. Give your health and your bank account a boost by drinking inexpensive, truly healthy natural spring water instead and getting your nutrients from food.

Unflavored, sugar and additive-free mineral water is also acceptable, particularly if it comes in glass rather than plastic bottles. Depending on where he lived, the Hunter would almost certainly have had access to and enjoyed mineral rich water sources in the wilderness. He and his family probably received a helpful nutrition boost from the minerals and trace minerals provided by this water source so, yes, feel free to enjoy mineral water. One word of caution though: Don't let mineral water become a replacement for pure, fresh water.

Water is by far the best and most Paleo-friendly beverage of all but if you are a lifelong soda or sweetened beverage drinker, you may find the switch to pure water a little daunting. If that's the case, please check out the awesome naturally flavored water recipes I've compiled for you in this book's recipe index. Thee fresh and juicy but still healthy drinks will help you change your drinking habits for the better in no time!

Dairy Beverages: Dairy beverages like milk, kefir and liquid yogurt drinks are often slightly controversial when it comes to their Paleo status. That's because some people argue that hunter-gatherers had no access to domesticated animals and so were not likely to be ingesting dairy products in any quantity. Other experts however, point out that while whole milk and fermented milk products were not necessarily a component of the earliest societies' diets, they do have an ancient and nutrient −rich basis in the human diet. They also say that milk is an important nourisher for humans at birth and through childhood and while it may not be required in large amounts after adulthood, it can and should form a limited part of a healthy primal diet. My stance on the dairy questions is simple: You know your body best. If you have no digestive, energy, mood or weight problems after consuming dairy products- by all means go ahead and include dairy in your Paleo life plan. If you do experience some symptoms after consuming milk, then, depending on the severity of those symptoms, you may want to consider cutting dairy out of your diet either permanently or for a while. If you aren't sure about how dairy affects your body, the best plan of action is to cut out all traces of dairy from your diet for a minimum of 30 days. Carefully note how you feel once dairy has been eliminated from your diet. Then, after the 30-day removal period, gradually add dairy back into your diet.

Again, carefully note how you feel after consuming dairy. If you find that negative symptoms arise, this could be a health wake-up call. Listen to your body. It will tell you very clearly if all dairy is fine, if only certain kinds of dairy are acceptable or if it needs you to eliminate all dairy sources for a while or permanently. There is no nutritionist, dietician, doctor or diet book that can take the place of actively observing your body's own reactions and learning from them.

Important Things to Think About When Selecting Dairy Beverages:

Pasteurization: Pasteurized milk is definitely NOT Paleo. This is because pasteurization is a modern invention that is supposedly "healthy" but in fact kills all of the nutritional value that milk has to offer your body. Regardless of whether you have any signs of lactose intolerance or not, pasteurization can make milk a major problem for your digestive system. This is because the precious enzymes that exist naturally in milk are completely ruined by pasteurization. Additionally, valuable vitamins such as vitamin C, B6, A and B12 are depleted and the healthy but very delicate proteins found in milk are transformed into strange, abnormal amino acid structures that your body does not and cannot recognize. Raw milk is also packed with highly useful and health-promoting bacteria but once pasteurized, these bacteria are destroyed. Pasteurization is the main culprit behind the idea that milk is somehow a threat to your well-being and is the reason why so many people are advised to give it a miss. My advice would be to try unpasteurized, raw milk before you decide on whether milk is or is not a beneficial part of your Paleo diet.

(Note: For a complete explanation of dairy issues and options, simply head to chapter 5 where I've discussed all things dairy in detail!)

Natural Dairy Substitutes: Many people these days feel that "natural" substitutes are better for you than animal products. To be clear, this usually goes against the very essence of the paleo plan. It is difficult (but not impossible!) to be truly Paleo while vegan because animal sources make up a large and very nutritious portion of the Paleo meal plan. However, when it comes to natural dairy substitutes, there are some options that are preferred:

Almond/Cashew Milk: We know that our hunter-gatherer ancestors had access to nuts but also that this access was very limited. Therefore, think quality over quantity when it comes to nuts in general and also when it comes to milk substitutes made from nuts. This means that almond milk, as long as it is chemical and additive –free, contains no sugar and is packaged in a plastic-free manner, can be an excellent addition to your warm morning drink of choice, cooked items or smoothies, in limited amounts. The main reason for the limitation stems from the fact that nuts tend to be higher in carbohydrates than the full-fat dairy products they are meant to replace and this can throw off your blood sugar. A central rule in the Paleo way of eating is the maintenance of an even and regulated blood glucose level and drinking or eating large doses of nut products could make it difficult to achieve the paleo results you're looking for.

Soy Milk: Soy milk is not considered Paleo. It is also not a healthy choice for any type of diet, for various reasons ranging from hormonal and thyroid disruption to anti-nutrient content. There is absolutely no reason to consume soymilk or any other non-organic and unfermented soy products. Soy is a highly estrogenic and carcinogenic substance and should not be consumed at all, on a healthy Paleo diet.

Coconut Milk: The coconut is a fantastic, fatty and all-natural fruit/pseudo-nut that Paleo people are free to include liberally into their diet. Because coconuts were available to many hunter-gatherer tribes in warmer climates and also because of their unprocessed, super-healthy, high-fat content, I advise making them a major part of your Paleo eating plan. Coconut milk, which comes from shredded coconut flesh, mixed with pure water and then squeezed through a strainer, is a rich, creamy and absolutely delicious dairy substitute for everything from warm beverages to smoothies as well as soups and sauces that require a rich "dairy" kick.

As an added bonus, coconuts are considered some of the most anti-inflammatory foods on Earth, making your Paleo eating plan a truly healing and revitalizing journey for your body!

Green Tea/ White Tea & Black Tea: Although not strictly caveman fare, tea can be an amazing addition to your healthy Paleo lifestyle. Its wonderful benefits often far outweigh any downsides and as long as the tea you select is natural, additive-free and prepared properly, it can help you to harness better health and even weight loss!

Tea is extremely anti-inflammatory and also offers major antioxidant benefits, which can help you to deal with and ward off many types of pains and ailments, from arthritis to cardiac inflammation and even Alzheimer's disease. Research overwhelmingly supports tea as a highly protective substance, helping to keep illnesses and conditions like high blood pressure, osteoporosis, cardiovascular diseases and even a range of cancers at bay. There has also been some preliminary research into findings that tea consumption could help to decrease how much carbohydrates your body absorbs! Tea has also been proven to play a major role in improving your body's ability to fight off a whole host of different bacterial infections.

Aside from this, its polyphenols have been linked to a marked anti-aging effect in regular consumers and it anecdotally has been believed to be a calming, stress-relieving substance.

Let's take a look at the various types of teas available to you on a Paleo Plan and how much of each type you should be consuming:

White Tea: White tea is basically tea in its rawest, most natural form. Because it is the least processed of all forms of tea, it is also the richest in health-boosting polyphenols. White tea also does not present the same tooth-staining problems posed by over-consumption of black teas, making it an excellent choice for those who want to reap all the rewards of tea without staining those pearly whites. Additionally, white tea provides your body with the lowest amount of caffeine, compared to other "true (non-herbal) teas" so if you're worried about caffeine intake, you can enjoy 2-3 cups of white tea per day, without concern.

Green Tea: Also less processed than traditional black tea, green tea offers you a wide and rich range of antioxidants, polyphenols and other health promoting substances. It has been researched for its purported, calming, clarity endowing and weight loss promoting benefits and many Paleo eaters choose it as a switch out for times when drinking just plain water isn't so appealing. Enjoy green tea warm with a dollop of raw honey or chilled with a wedge of lemon and a couple of ice cubes. It makes for a great, natural energy booster in place of the sugary, chemical-laden energy and sports drinks that are just not Paleo. Add more lemon into your cool green tea if you are using it as a sports drink as the lemon will give your drink an added potassium boost(way more than Gatorade, for example)and help to replace precious electrolytes lost during exercise.

Black Tea: One of the most ancient and beloved beverages worldwide, black tea offers numerous health benefits to back up its popularity. It provides your body with cholesterol-lowering effects as well as easing blood pressure and improving blood circulation. It also benefits your digestion, decreases diarrhea, prevents tooth decay and bacterial infections, has upper-respiratory protective effects and can even improve asthma. Because black tea undergoes a mild fermentation process, it also provides benefits from a fermented foods angle and is widely used in Asian cooking as well as medicinal tonic making.

According to numerous studies, black tea can provide far-reaching cardiovascular benefits, currently unequalled by other beverages. Because cardiovascular disease is the number one killer, adding black tea into your diet in amounts of up to 3 cups daily can be a smart move that increases your chances of being a healthy hunter and not the prey to modern diseases.

Herbal Teas: While not "true teas" and lacking the huge antioxidant and polyphenol content provided in black, green, oolong and white teas, herbal teas can offer you a range of effective health promoting bonuses. Because wild herbs grew in most environments, were often gathered by our hunter-gatherer ancestors and may have even boiled up into soothing and medicinal drinks, you can be sure that adding herbal teas into your Paleo diet is a good and truly primal idea. Whether you choose mint for its digestive system aiding properties or lemongrass for its zing and delicate flavor, turmeric for anti-pain and anti-inflammatory abilities or cumin for its fresh taste and brain-function promoting powers, you can enjoy a wide range of herbal teas freely, as long as you don't add sugar to your beverages. Instead, add a small amount of raw honey (not more than once a day), a little stevia (if it suits you) or even a couple of sticks of cinnamon for natural sweetness that also curbs sugar cravings.

Coffee: This is a hot topic in the Paleo community and rightly so. Millions of people worldwide would not dream of starting their day off without a warm, steaming brew of aromatic coffee. While we know our Paleo ancestors didn't have access to coffee (just like they definitely weren't brewing up pots of green, black or white tea by the cooking fire!), the many health benefits of this remarkable drink make it a beverage many Paleo eaters choose to include in their Paleo eating plans and lifestyle. Let's take a look at some of the most astonishing bonuses in that steaming mug of coffee:

Research shows that regular consumption of coffee is closely linked to having lower body weight and lower rates of type 2 diabetes.

Drinking coffee has also been linked to lower rates of non-alcoholic fatty liver disease. Coffee is also loaded with those same heart-healthy, anti-aging and disease preventative antioxidants and polyphenols that make drinking tea such a great idea. In fact, coffee has proven to be so beneficial that when overweight individuals were instructed to drink large amounts of coffee their liver function markers showed improvements in testing and their supply of adipose tissue also showed enhanced functioning!

With all of that being said, however, there are some important factors to remember to make sure that your cup of coffee (or 2!) is aiding your Paleo lifestyle fully:

Limit your consumption of carbohydrate rich foods when drinking coffee: If you are looking for a quick breakfast to cushion your stomach with your morning coffee, DON'T go for carb-heavy meals or ultra-sweet fruits! Improve your insulin sensitivity while enjoying your coffee by pairing your beverage with foods rich in proteins and fats like eggs, bacon or other fatty meats or organ meats. A great, highly–effective, energy boosting and extremely affordable breakfast option is a nice cup of black coffee and a handful of grilled or sautéed kidneys with onions! Try this combo once and you'll absolutely keep coming back for more!

Don't stay stationary after enjoying your coffee break: because coffee has the ability to free a large amount of fatty acids from your body's store of adipose tissue, it is very important to utilize these freed fatty acids properly. If you stay stationary after your cup of coffee, you risk allowing these fatty acids being replaced right back into your adipose tissue. The best way to make the most of your afternoon coffee break is to take a stroll around the office, head to the parking lot for a brisk walk or do leg and arm exercises t your desk. If you drink coffee in the mornings, try to time your morning cup to coincide with your early morning workout. Using those freed fatty acids will help you to make the most of coffee's weight-lowering effects and also reduce any caffeine jitters!

Don't binge on any beverage calories to the detriment of food calories: As Paleo eaters, we seek to emulate the lifestyles and eating patterns of our early hunter-gatherer ancestors. This means eating and NOT drinking the bulk of our caloric intake for the day. Many Americans now consume a huge portion of their daily calories in drink forms ranging from fruit juices and sodas to coffees and smoothies. It is very important that you avoid this way of drinking at all costs. While drinking a couple of mugs of coffee is not a problem and can in fact be highly beneficial to your Paleo lifestyle, don't mistake this for an excuse to add loads of sugar, unnatural flavors and additives to your cup.

Your coffee should be as natural as possible, sourced from good quality Arabica beans and ground at home or by a retailer you can trust not to add gluten, grain additives and chemical flavors to your blend. You can add full-fat dairy in the form of unpasteurized milk, heavy cream or even raw, organic, grass-fed sourced butter into your cup for a healthy, creamy and delicious treat but absolutely avoid all low-fat, skim and non-dairy chemical additives. You can also use coconut milk or oil blended into your coffee for a non-animal fat, but still totally Paleo enhancer. When it comes to sweetening, aim for no sugar, a little stevia or raw honey or even cinnamon to give you subtle sweetness that won't take you away from your paleo roots.

Now that we've got the coffee question solved, head to the next chapter where we look at Paleo beverages part 2 for even more useful and cost-effective Paleo drink information!

Chapter 12:
Paleo Beverages Part 2: What's In, What's Out and How to Decide

In the last chapter, we looked at largely beneficial drinks like water, coffee, tea ,coconut milk and others as well as how to consume them properly in a Paleo format. Let's take a look now at drinks that are definitely NOT Paleo and should be totally avoided!

Commercial Fruit Juices: Don't let the pictures and seemingly healthy names fool you, the majority of commercially available fruit juices are actually just fruit-flavored sugary syrups that will do absolutely nothing good for your body. While our hunter-gatherer ancestors certainly had access to and enjoyed wild fruits and vegetables in their purest and freshest forms, the fruit juices lining the aisles of today's supermarkets are completely different from real fruit. Bottled or otherwise packaged fruit juices are frequently filled with preservatives and additives that are toxic and foreign to your body's digestive system, while the packaging they come in often contains BPA plastics or other harmful materials that are endocrine-disruptors. If you think that's not enough to steer clear of these so-called fruit juices, then consider this: All those vitamins advertised on the back of those juice bottle sand jugs are actually artificially added to the juice AFTER the production process. The naturally occurring vitamins that make fruit such an important part of a healthy diet are nowhere to be found. This is because when these commercially prepared fruit juices are exposed to oxygen, the precious vitamin content that fruits provide is quickly destroyed. Manufacturers know that you drink fruit juice because it is a good source of vitamins and minerals so they then go in and "doctor" this nutritionally dead juice by fortifying it with artificially added vitamins and minerals. In the process, the fruit juice is leached of its important fibers and turned into a sugary, insulin-raising product that wreaks havoc on your body's delicately balanced blood glucose levels!

If you want to reap all of the health (and flavor) rewards of fruits, then consume them in the way your body was naturally meant to enjoy them- with all of their fiber content and in some cases with their peel intact. Make your own fresh-squeezed juices at home (not too frequently, remember, we aim to eat, not drink, our calories.) and load up on the juicy pulp and skins when it comes to smoothies.

Think about it, the Hunter definitely didn't have the time or the inclination to go around discarding precious sources of nutrition like the fibrous parts of fruit or removing any edible skin from them. If you're a fan of peeling apples or removing the skin from your grapes before juicing, remember that you are also removing a vital source of fiber and many polyphenols and nutrients that can help your body to utilize the fruit you're consuming in the best possible way.

The Paleo verdict on commercially available fruit juice: Ditch the artificial flavorings, colors and chemicals and opt for real fruit juice made at home (or at a juice bar you can trust not to add flavors or preservatives) instead.

Soda: Soda is literally and nutritionally at the bottom of the list when it comes to beverages. The human body derives absolutely no benefit from consuming soda and instead, is exposed to an extremely frightening array of health threats and dangers after only a couple of sips of this sickly sweet poison. So exactly what is it about soda that makes it just about the unhealthiest thing you can put into your body? A single can of soda contains 16 entire cubes of sugar! Soda is so easy to drink that swallowing down a whole can in just a couple of minutes is no difficult task. This is why frequently drinking soda leads to a scarily rapid spike in blood sugar, completely destroying your body's insulin regulating mechanisms. Regular consumption of soft drinks is concretely linked to a massively increased risk of developing type 2 diabetes.

It was virtually unknown in the ancient world of hunter-gatherers and yet today, type2 diabetes is one of the fastest growing risks facing the global population as it brings with a whole host of destructive conditions, from cardiovascular disease to liver, kidney and pancreatic failure, nerve damage and the permanent destruction of brain matter. If only one disease could be the poster child for the failures of modern eating, it would be type 2 diabetes hands down.

Soda also contains dangerous artificial coloring and flavoring agents like the chemical4-methylimidazole, a lethal carcinogen that gives soda that alluring caramel color. Recent research points to an increased risk of developing cancer from consuming the amount of 4-methylimidazole in just one can of soda. Regular soft drink consumers are at a higher risk for developing a range of deadly cancers, including colon, esophageal, liver and breast cancer so stay away from soda if you want to enjoy the health and vitality of your hunter-gatherer ancestors!

Soda is doing you no favors when it comes to your brain either. Consuming soft drink scan destroy your brain's natural ability to create new brain cells and make new information and learning-boosting pathways. Every time you take a sip of the toxic brew in a soda can, you are drastically reducing your brain's ability to adapt to new situations, to learn and retain new information and to fend off the accumulation of plaque. Plaque deposits in the brain have been directly linked to the development of terrifying degenerative diseases like Parkinson's and Alzheimer's disease. These types of diseases didn't affect our ancient ancestors but our modern ways of eating and drinking have led them to become a rapidly expanding problem in our times.

Diet Soda: What about diet soda, you may be wondering? Isn't it much safer than regular soda? The short and definitive answer to that question is a resounding NO! Just in case you're at all unclear about this, let me just say that if you're ever in the position of having to choose a soda drink, please make sure that you go for a can of regular instead of diet. This is because diet soda, although stripped of the sugar that regular soda contains, is actually a much more deadly drink than any variety of regular soda. Let's look at some of the toxic effects of diet soda:

Because diet soda is meant to be a sugar-free alternative to regular soda's whopping sugar content, it is flavored through the addition of artificial sweeteners such as aspartame and sucralose. Let's look at these two known neurotoxins:

Aspartame: The consumption of aspartame has been linked to a long list of health problems from headaches and migraines to a variety of cancers. Aspartame is a mix of isolated, dangerous amino acids and wood alcohol and has been shown in tests to damage brain cells and destroy beneficial gut flora.

Sucralose: Sucralose is a synthetic organochlorine compound that is chemically similar to deadly pesticides such as DDT and PCBs. It is both a known endocrine disruptor and a carcinogen. It is a ridiculous 600 times more sweet than natural sugar but its effects on the body are nothing to savor!

Diet soda also contains phosphoric acid, a type of acid that is cheaper to manufacture than the previously used citric acid and has much worse effects. Phosphoric acid is infamous for stripping calcium stores from your bones, decreasing the mineral density of your bones and leading to osteoporosis.

If all of the symptoms and disease above aren't enough to convince you that diet soda doesn't deserve a place in your fridge or your body, perhaps this will: Studies have shown time and time again that although the soda is called "diet" it actually leads to increased rates of weight gain. In fact, regular consumption of diet soda is linked to rising risk for obesity and the MORE so-called diet soda your drink, the MORE you actually set yourself up for stubborn weight gain. Take a leaf from the Hunter's book and only consume drinks that exist in nature. If you want to eat like the victor and not the victim, kick all of those cans of soft drinks to the curb for good and embrace healthy Paleo options like natural mineral water and teas instead.

Chapter 13:
Real Food for Real Health: A Definitive List of No-Paleo Food Additives to Avoid

The Hunter was always on the lookout for nutrient-rich, fresh and vital sources of food and to access the very best results of the Paleo way of eating, we should be following his lead. This means including nutritious eats, seafood, fats, vegetables, fruits, nuts and seeds to our diets. What it definitely doesn't mean is including processed, chemical-laden, high preservative, high additive "Franken-foods" that are more of a science experiment than a source of nourishment for human beings.

To put my point very simply, the foods we should be avoiding generally do not grow in the wild but instead, come wrapped up in shiny packages, bottles, cans and brightly colored boxes and bags. They are much more likely to give us an unnecessary and harmful dose of chemicals than they are to give us any level of beneficial nutrition. The best and easiest way to avoid these foods is to shop for whole, real foods as close to their natural state as possible. You can do this by shopping the perimeters of your local grocery store and giving the central aisles, where all of the packaged, processed horrors lurk, a wide berth. But sometimes it becomes a necessity to venture beyond the produce, meats, seafood and dairy sections. In fact, more than 75 percent of all supermarket shelf space is taken up by chemically processed foods and in the US, more than 3000 different kinds of additives are regularly added to common foods! That's why a thorough guide to the non-Paleo additives to avoid comes in handy and for that reason, I've compiled an in-depth list of additives to look out for and additives to completely avoid. So put those ancient survival skills to good use and keep your eyes open for any of these toxic threats to your health and weight loss, on your next shopping trip: Happy hunting!

Here are some of the top additives to watch out for:

1. **Nitrates:** Nitrates are added to processed meats in order to add color (giving that bright red color to hams, hot dogs and bacon), enhance flavor and extend their life-span. While many people believe sodium nitrate is safe and just a form of "salt", it was considered so dangerous that it was nearly banned from the food supply in the 1970's. This is because nitrates are well-known

carcinogens, creating compounds called nitrosamines. Nitrosamines are cancer-causing and are behind the rise in stomach and colorectal cancers in people who regularly consume processed meat. Nitrosamines are especially dangerous in the case of high-heat cooking, so throwing those hot dogs on the grill can make their nitrate content even more carcinogenic!

Nitrates are Usually Found In:

- **Ham**

- **Bacon**

- **Sausages**

- **Hot Dogs**

- **Corned Beef**

- **And Any Other Smoked or Processed Meats**

This doesn't mean that you cannot enjoy a Paleo full fat bacon breakfast. Simply look for nitrate-free bacon and you're good to go!

2. **Artificial Coloring (Caramel Coloring):** You'll find caramel coloring

listed on the back of many foods and beverages as artificial color. This coloring agent is used to give many foods and drinks an appealing golden brown hue but its health effects ae not as attractive: Caramel coloring has been proven in tests to increase the risk of cancer, due to its byproduct 4-Methylimidazole (4-Mel).

Caramel Coloring is Usually Found In:

- **Baked Goods**

- **Sodas**

- **Diet Sodas**

- **Coffee and Caramel "flavored" Drinks and Desserts**

- **Snack Items**

3. **Top Food Dyes:** While there are 9 different kinds of food dyes commonly in use, these are the major ones to watch out for:

Red 40, (allura red AC): Contains the known carcinogen p-Cresidine.

Yellow 5: Associated to ADD-like symptoms and hyperactivity, problems focusing in children. Contains the known carcinogen benzidine, 4-amino-biphenyl

Yellow 6: Contains the known carcinogen benzidine, 4-amino-biphenyl

These dyes are mainly derived from petroleum or coal sources and pose a serious risk of cancer development.

These Top Food Dyes are Usually Found In:

- **Cereals**

- **Candies**

- **Snacks**

- **Fruit Juices**

- **Sodas**

- **Energy Drinks**

- **Flavored Chips**

- **And Many Other Food and Drink Items**

Because these food dyes are so dangerous and prevalent make sure you examine all food and beverage labels for them, before consuming.

4. Propyl Gallate

Propyl gallate is added to food to lengthen its sell-by date and to keep the fats found in many foods from spoiling naturally. Propyl gallate is another sneaky additive that's potentially harmful. This additive can cause hormonal imbalances, particularly in women, causing lowered estrogen production. It has also been shown to be linked to possible cancer-development.

Propyl Gallate is Usually Found In:

- **Snacks**

- **Oils**

- **Meats**

- **Soup Mixes**

- **Potato Chips**

- **Chewing Gums**

5. BHT (Butylated Hydroxytoluene):
Yet another great reason to avoid all processed foods is BHT. This additive is found both in many food items AND in embalming fluids, jet fuel, petroleum products and even transformer oil. This additive is beloved by food manufacturers who utilize it to add color, enhance flavor and make food items last way beyond their natural shelf-life. BHT is a carcinogen that can cause severe harm to the liver and possibly other organs:

BHT Is Usually Found In:

- **Snack Items**

- **Candy**

- **Chewing Gum**

- **Breakfast Cereals**

- **Lard (Lard is not a great Paleo Source of Fat!)**

- **Shortening**

- **Meats**

- **Oils**

6. **MSG (Monosodium Glutamate):** **MSG** (Monosodium glutamate) is an additive that is widely used in many food items in order to adjust flavor and preserve the products for long term use. MSG has been proven to make the body more susceptible to the development and growth of cancer. MSG has also nee linked with a rise in chronic inflammation and obesity. Consumers have voiced their concerns over the use of MSG so now it is very unlikely that you will see the actual "MSG" label on any products. Instead, it lurks inside processed foods under these numerous guises:

MSG Is Often Labeled As:

- Carrageenan

- Autolyzed yeast

- Disodium inosinate

- Maltodextrin

- Hydrolyzed soy protein

- Textured soy protein concentrate

- Modified Cornstarch

- Disodium Guaylate

MSG is Usually Found In:

- **Potato Chips**

- **Snack Items**

- **Sauces**

- **Seasonings**

- **Cookies**

- **Soup Mixes**

- **Lunch Meats**

- **Dairy Items (Cheeses, Fat-Free or Low-Fat Milk, Ice Cream, Powdered Milk)**

- Baby Formulas

- Infant Foods

MSG can hide in some of the most unlikely places so extreme vigilance is necessary. Don't just assume that any processed food is MSG-free because the MSG label is nowhere in sight. As you can see, MSG comes in many, many different forms and can be added into even health-minded products, so keep your eyes open and when in doubt, skip that food or beverage. Also, if you find yourself developing a headache or rash regularly after consuming a certain product, there is a good chance that you are experiencing an MSG-reaction. Eliminate that item from your diet because it is always better to be safe (and truly Paleo) than sorry!

7. **Sweeteners:** Artificial sweetening agents such as aspartame and sucralose are in wide spread use as many manufacturers aim to provide lots of "low-sugar" and "sugar-free" items to the public. However, these sweetening agents are in many cases much worse than pure table sugar because of their serious health effects.

Aspartame: While many manufacturers insist that aspartame is 100 percent safe, anecdotal and research results tell us differently. Just like MSG, aspartame is believed to be Aspartame an "excitotoxin". Excitotoxins are neurotoxins, compounds that are known to Over-excite the brains nerve cells and lead to inability to concentrate, anxiety and even cognitive decline.

Aspartame also poses a huge health risk to those who are unable to properly metabolize a substance in aspartame called phenylalanine. Those with the genetic disorder phenylketonuria (PKU) suffer from these harmful effects. Those who are pregnant and have an abundance of phenylalanine in their blood streams as well as those suffering from liver disease can end up with serious damage to the brain after consuming aspartame.

Aspartame Must Be Labelled in The US and is Often Found In:

- **Diet Products**

- **Sugar-Free Sodas and Drinks**

- **Low-Sugar and No-Sugar Desserts**

Sucralose: This artificial sweetening agent provides a whopping 600 times the sweetness of natural sugar! And that unnatural sweetness comes with serious side effects. Research has linked sucralose to an increased risk of leukemia development in regular users. Studies also indicate that sucralose alters glucose and insulin, leading to type 2 diabetes, obesity and insulin resistance.

Splenda Is Also Usually Found In:

- **Diet Products**

- **Sugar-Free Sodas and Drinks**

- **Low-Sugar and No-Sugar Desserts**

Real Food for Real Results: Paleo at Its Most Natural

Paleo is considered one of the cleanest ways of eating possible because it follows one basic principle: The natural, ancestral and intuitive ways of eating that have been the mainstay of humanity for millennia.

When you are eating in a Paleo way, you are consuming mostly the same whole, real, healthy foods that our ancestor the Hunter would have craved and recognized, ensuring that your body does not suffer from the many additives and unknown chemicals being poured into processed "fake" foods today. On those rare occasions when you have no access to real foods, you may be forced to choose something processed. In such a case, reading all labels and choosing the item that does not include these dangerous additives is your best bet to protect your body and brain from the many lethal poisons that are "legally" edible in modern foods.

Chapter 13:
The Autoimmune Paleo Protocol:
An Ancient Cure for Modern-Day
Conditions (Part 1)

Are you on one of the millions of people around the world whose body is battling against you? Do you suffer from the ravages of autoimmune conditions such a fibromyalgia, multiple sclerosis, HS, lupus or rheumatoid arthritis among many others? If so, this chapter on the Autoimmune Paleo Protocol is just for you. The Autoimmune Paleo Protocol (AIP for short), is a way of eating that is Paleo but has been further adjusted to bring all of the healing benefits of the Paleo diet to those suffering from the silent but deadly havoc that autoimmune diseases can wreak on the body, mind, mood and life.

When you have an autoimmune diseases or disorder, it can be very difficult to see yourself as anything other than a victim. That's because these conditions are so tough to even diagnose, let alone alleviate or treat. Conventional medicine likes to throw pills at any condition it doesn't fully understand and the problem with that is, often times these pills are, at best, nothing more than bandages over gaping wounds and at worst, toxic chemical concoctions that can cause your condition to go south faster than simply leaving yourself untreated. When faced with such a choice, many autoimmune sufferers simply end up feeling despondent and "beyond help". But I'm here to tell you that this is absolutely not true. There are ways to treat and even send autoimmune disorders into long term remission, without the use of harsh prescription drugs, endless, expensive doctor's appointments and unhelpful diets. These ways are as old as humanity itself, because they are rooted in the ways humans have always eaten. They are based on the natural gifts of nutrition and these nourishing ways can help to slow down, then reduce and ultimately eliminate the activities of autoimmune conditions within your body. Without further ado, let's jump in and get started! After all, the sooner the healing starts, the sooner you can begin to feel better and return to enjoying your daily life:

Understanding Autoimmune Disease

Autoimmune disease is a condition characterized by the body being unable to differentiate between its own healthy tissue and dangerous foreign substances invading it. When this occurs, the body becomes extremely sensitive and launches a full-scale attack against the "foreign invaders" which are in reality, its own healthy, harmless tissues. This process of battling its own bodily tissues can start slowly and grow in scale and ferocity over many months and even years! While this is taking place, you may feel more tired than usual, slightly feverish, cloudy and confused but you will likely have no idea that a vicious battle is taking place inside your body and that you have in essence, become the victim of your own over-zealous and befuddled immune system. At some stage in this process, your hypersensitivity develops into an actual autoimmune disease or disorder. It is important to note that while, at current count, there are over 80 different, officially recognized autoimmune disorders and that even more are being pinpointed and labelled as you read this, all autoimmune disorders are actually very closely related. They are all highly inflammatory, and are all centered on this confusion of the autoimmune system and the resulting war against your own body. With all autoimmune disorders, your brain tissue, thyroid gland tissue, salivary gland tissue, the collage in your skin and between your joints, your tendons and even your digestive organs and lung tissue, all generally come under fire from your over active immune system. This is precisely why autoimmune sufferers so often complain that it "hurts everywhere". One of the rules of medicine that conventional Western doctors usually standby is that when a patient complains of pain everywhere, that means it's a psychosomatic or imagined ailment. Many times, sufferers of autoimmune disorders fail to get a proper diagnosis because conventional doctors tell them that it is impossible to be in pain "everywhere". And yet, we know that autoimmune disorders blindly attack all kinds of tissue in the bodies of these patients, often simultaneously, and that their feelings of generalized pain ARE NOT imagined!

The Autoimmune Paleo Protocol (AIP)

That's where the Autoimmune Paleo Protocol comes in. In the face of unsuitable ineffective and sometimes even harmful treatments for autoimmune conditions, many sufferers have begun to adopt a new way of eating that in reality is the most ancient and authentic way of eating there is. The have found that food truly is medicine and that the Paleo diet has radically transformed the way they feel, perform and live on a day-to-day basis. However, when it comes to autoimmune disorders, the body is in a hypersensitive, hyper-alert and irritated state and whereas the average healthy person can adopt simple Paleo practices wholesale and see amazing results, those with autoimmune disorders do need to be cautious with certain aspects of their diet. That's why the AIP is specifically altered to suit the needs of those with autoimmune disorders.

Heal the Gut, Heal the Body

The main aim of the Autoimmune Paleo Protocol (AIP) diet is to cool, heal and treat any inflammation within the digestive system, specifically the intestines. A large portion of autoimmune sufferers are on elimination diets or have tried them at some stage because they are so widely known to have a positive effect on autoimmune conditions. However, the standard elimination diets out there usually only provide very limited effects because they are themselves, rather limited in scope. The AIP diet goes far beyond these standard elimination diets, to successfully wipe out the foods and substances that signal and start the chronic fire of inflammation within the gut and then the entire body. Because the AIP eliminates these threats and irritants, it allows the gut to begin to heal, seal up and cool while also giving the rest of your body a chance to recuperate from the inflammation that has spread around it from the gut. In order to understand how this works, let's take a look at what are commonly called the "three brains": the gut, the skin and the brain.

The Gut-Skin-Brain Connection: How the AIP Can Heal the "Three Brains":

Many people believe that their moods and cognitive functions are regulated by their mind, while their digestive processes are governed by their guts and the state of their complexions, the production of natural oils, and the ability to keep harmful dermal conditions away are all controlled by their skin. Well, this has been the prevailing school of thought for many decades but the truth is that the human body is an incredibly complex, integrated and inter-linked organism. It is not possible to break up certain functions and processes into small compartments and claim that they are only affected by one area of the body, while others are regulated by another part. In short, there is very little division between our body's functions and the sooner we realize the extent to which all functions are affected by all parts of us, the better we can treat and prevent conditions like autoimmune disorders that seem to "spread" throughout every part of the body.

We call this theory of inter-linkage the "three brains theory" because it is becoming ever clearer that the human body's functions are regulated, ruled and balanced by three main areas: Our guts, our brains and our skin! To understand this, we have to hark back to groundbreaking research done by various scientists and dermatologists such as Donald M. Pillsbury and John H. Stokes. This research uncovered a link or overlapping between the disturbances of the gut such as indigestion and constipation, disturbances of the mind such as anxiety disorders and depression and disturbances of the skin such as acne and irritation. So how does this work? Acute emotional stress triggers an avalanche of negative effects on the health of gut bacteria. When the distress of the mind leads to the die off large quantities of good bacteria in the gut, bad bacteria allow the gut to become inflamed, fragile and permeable. Leaky gut syndrome ensues and this permeability allows dangerous substances to leak out of the gut, into the blood stream setting off a series of systemic inflammatory conditions and resulting in, among other things, acne, skin irritations and lesions, more depression and stress . The more stress and depression occur, the more the gut again becomes inflamed and the whole cycle continues viciously and unbreakably.

This school of thought has gained ground with proof that over 40 percent of all acne sufferers in one study were found to have low levels of stomach acid production. This insufficiency caused dangerous bacteria to move up from the lower gastrointestinal tract (for example: the colon) where they usually resided, into the upper GI tract where they definitely do not belong. This sudden arrival of unfamiliar bad bacteria completely destroyed the delicate balance of good bacteria in the gut microbiome and led to the inflammation and permeability of the gut, which itself led to the emergence of these skin conditions.

Other studies also show us that there are unusually low levels of positive good bacteria within the feces of those suffering with various mental and psychiatric disorders, proving further the link between the body's three brains: the gut, the skin and the brain.

So how does this affect autoimmune sufferers? Well, we are now seeing the poisonous fruits of our shift away from the natural, ancestral, healing Paleo ways of eating. We have left behind the wise and nourishing food habits that mankind has always practiced. Our new, modern, commercialized and heavily processed diets are completely destroying our digestive systems and leading to unnatural, imbalanced gut biomes in which good bacteria are dying off and bad bacteria are flourishing, all at the expense of our health, well-being and even our sanity.

As a consequence of these shortsighted actions on our part, we are now in the midst of a literal tidal wave of autoimmune disorders and diseases, the likes of which have never been seen or experienced by humanity before! These autoimmune disorders start very slowly and surreptitiously, taking the guise of gastrointestinal problems including constipation, diarrhea, Irritable Bowel Syndrome (IBS), nausea and acid reflux. It is a well-known fact that such gastrointestinal issues often bring with them a whole host of emotional and mental disturbances from panic attacks and general anxiety to depression and an inability to concentrate. With such emotional and mental disturbances come another set of problems this time affecting the skins health and appearance. These include redness, irritation, dermatitis and severe cases of acne vulgaris.

In fact, a condition closely tied with autoimmune disorders of all kinds, called SIBO (Small Intestinal Bacterial Overgrowth), actually comes from an insufficient level of stomach acid production. This low level of stomach acid causes the overgrowth of bad bacteria (hence the name of the condition) and can present in a wide range of ways, from extreme bloating and swelling to the inability to absorb nutrients such as vitamin B, which are essential for mental health and mood regulation. SIBO is often found in those suffering with autoimmune disorders such as chronic fatigue syndrome, thyroid disorders and fibromyalgia, so if you have or suspect you have any of these disorders, it would be highly advisable to get your stool checked out medically to find out whether or not you have an overgrowth of bad bacteria within your system.

How The Autoimmune Paleo Protocol (AIP) Can Heal The Total Body Through The "Three Brains":

Because nutrition affects your entire body, the AIP is a total body plan. It works in an integrative way to address the interlinked issues in the three brains of the gut, skin and brain, setting the stage for the healing of all parts of the body where the systemic inflammation of autoimmune disorders causes damage and destruction.

The AIP diets primary focus is on repairing the damage done to the digestive system specifically the intestinal lining, the balance of gut microflora and the intestinal mucosa, while at the same time providing nutritional support that can decrease the amount of chronic inflammation throughout the body. In this way, your body gets the opportunity to begin to heal while the AIP diet ensures that no irritants are consumed that could lead to another flare-up of the autoimmune condition. The AIP is a long term plan that teaches you to eat and live in a balanced and healing way but really, it is an ancient and ancestral eating plan that human beings instinctively crave and thrive on because it is our most natural way of eating and living.

Starting the AIP: Phase 1-Elimination

Duration: 7-8 Weeks

The Following Foods Should Be Completely Eliminated For the Next 7 to 8 Weeks of Your AIP Diet:

- All Types of Legumes (Beans, Peas etc.)

- All Forms of Grains

- All Forms of Alternative Sweetening Agents Such as Stevia, Xylitol and Mannitol

- All Dried Fruits

- Limit Consumption of Fresh Fruits to No More than 2 Pieces Per Day

- All Dairy Products(You May Be Able to Tolerate and Add Fermented Dairy Back in During the Reintroduction Phase)

- All Nuts and Nut Oils

- All Tapioca and Tapioca Products(Can Often Cross-React With Gluten)

- All Seeds (Eliminate Chia Seeds, Flax Seeds, Sunflower Seeds, Sesame Seeds, Pumpkin Seeds as Well as Coriander Seeds and Cumin Seeds and Any Other Types of Seeds or Seed Products)

- Eggs(Neither Free-Range Nor Commercial Types Allowed for This Phase)

- Gums (Even Natural Types)

- All Processed and Packaged Foods

- All Forms of Alcohol

- All Types of Vegetable Oils (Permitted Oils Include Red Palm Oils, Olive Oil, Grass-Fed Ghee and Pure Coconut Oil)

- All Chocolate and Chocolate Products

- All Members of the Nightshade Plant Family Including Potatoes, Tomatoes, Peppers, Bell Peppers, Paprika, Mustard Seed, Egg Plant and All Pepper Products

- All Cooking Herbs that Come From Seeds

The Following Foods May Be Eaten Freely During the Elimination Phase and Beyond:

- Fresh Fruits (In Amounts of 2 Pieces Per Day)

- All Non-Nightshade Vegetables

- All Fats Such as Lard, Grass-Fed Beef Tallow, Bacon(Non-Nitrate) Fats, Cultured Grass-Fed Ghee Pure Olive and Coconut Oils

- All Fermented Foods Such as Fermented Vegetables(Kimchi without Eliminated Spices and Vegetables), Kombucha, Fermented Coconut Products

- Bone Broths

- Pure Beef Gelatin

- Pure Arrowroot Gelatin (If Tolerated)

- Vinegars(All Pure Vinegars Such as Balsamic and Apple Cider Allowed)

- Non-Fermented Pure Coconut Products(Except for Nectars and Sugars)

- Fresh and Frozen Non-Additive, Non-Processed Meats

- Fresh and Frozen Non-Additive, Non-Processed Poultry

- All Seafood(Wild-Caught is Best, Even if Frozen)

- Herbal and Green Teas (No Seed Teas Allowed)

- Pure Natural Sweeteners Such as Real Maple and Raw Honey Herbs in Amounts of No More Than 1 ½ Teaspoons Per Day

- All Freshly Ground Herbs (Only Non-Seed herbs)

Special FODMAPS Elimination Tip: If You Have a Known or Suspected Intolerance to High FODMAPS Foods, Please Also Remove All FODMAPS Foods From Your Diet During the Initial 7-8 Week Elimination Phase!

Methods For the Reintroduction Phase (To Be Done After Initial 7-8 Week Elimination Phase Has Been Successfully Completed)

- Only practice reintroduction of a new food once every 5 days. Begin By eating a small bite of the food. A few hours later, consume a larger bite and follow up by a full-sized serving. Remain vigilant for any changes or severe reactions.

- Reactions can emerge within a 72 hour window. It can take up to 3 days for your body to create IgA, IgG or IgM antibodies and for these antibodies to cause a noticeable reaction. For this reason, keep your eyes peeled for any symptoms within a 3 day window reintroducing an eliminated food. Look for symptoms such as fatigue, muscle and joint aches, indigestion and stomach pains, bloating, confusion and cloudy thinking, constipation, diarrhea or the inability to sleep well.

- Write down all symptoms reactions or lack of reactions in a dedicated journal. This will allow you to keep track of your progress during the reintroduction phase.

- Use the elimination phase not just to find out which foods you are most sensitive to, but also as a way to rest and cleanse your system periodically. In order to do this, schedule an elimination diet a couple of times a year to re-set your whole body and rebalance your good gut bacteria.

Chapter 14:
Using the Anti-Candida Diet to Deal Autoimmune Disorders the Final Blow! (Part 2)

After the initial eliminate and reintroduction phases are complete, you are very likely to see good results in terms of increased good gut microflora, decreased evidence of pathogenic bacteria and higher energy levels. However, for many people, a systemic candida infestation is at the root of their autoimmune disorder's emergence. If you find that you are still suffering from fatigue, weight gain, headaches and recurring yeast infections, candida may be to blame. Therefore, a full no-yeast, anti-candida diet may be indicated.

An Effective Anti-Candida Diet

Avoid:

- All Grains: Including Wheat, Oats, Barely, Rye, Spelt, Teff and All Products Made with Grains such as Breads, Pastas etc.

- All Corn and Corn Products

- All Rice and Rice Products

- Sugar

- Fructose

- High Fructose Corn Syrup

- Honey

- Syrups

- Rice Syrups

- All Artificial Sweeteners

- Chocolate

- Molasses

All Fruits Including:

- Fresh Fruit

- Canned Fruit

- Dried Fruit

- Fruit Juices

- Fruit Extracts

- Small Amounts of Lemon and Lime Are Allowed!

All Types of Alcohol:

- Beer

- Cider

- Wine

- Spirits

- Liquors

Beverages:

- Coffee

- Black Tea

- Green Tea

- Diet Soda

- Regular Soda

- Fruit Juices

- Energy Drinks

Vegetables:

- Peas

- Parsnips

- Potatoes

- Sweet Potatoes

- Yams

- Carrots

- Beets

Meats:

- Cured Meat

- Processed Meats

- Smoked Meats

- Pork and Pork Products

Shellfish and Fish:

- Packed, Cured or Canned Sardines

- All Types of Shellfish (All Types of Shellfish are Common Allergens)

Dairy:

Avoid All Dairy Such as:

- Cheese

- Milk

- Whey

- Cream

- Kefir, Live Yogurt and Raw Milk Butter Are All Allowed!

Condiments and Sauces:

- Ketchup

- Soy Sauce

- Regular Mustard

- Mayonnaise

- Horseradish

- Relish

- Avoid All Commercially Prepared Dressings and Sauces. Use Lemon Juice and Olive Oil Instead!

Oils:

- Canola Oil

- Corn Oil

- Soy Oil

- Peanut Oil

- Most of these Oils Are Contaminated with Mold and Can Feed Candida!

- Avoid All Legumes

- Avoid All Soy Products

- Avoid All Mushrooms and Fungi

- Avoid All Nuts-Many Contain Mold

- Avoid Additives, Preservatives and Chemicals- Eat Only Whole Natural Foods

- Avoid All Vinegar- Only Apple Cider Vinegar is Allowed!

Natural Anti-Candida Supplementation:

Depending on the severity of your case of candida, you may need to remain on this diet for a minimum of 2-4 months. In that time, all traces of systemic candida will be starved of all the foods and beverages that regularly feed it and will die off. In order to encourage this die-off, there are several very important, powerful natural supplements that can weaken and help to eliminate candida from your body completely:

Natural Olive Leaf Extract: Natural olive leaf extract has been found in several studies as well as anecdotally to be effective against candida, even when medications fail. Oleuropein is the active ingredient found in olive leaf extract and it is this ingredient that is capable of wiping out candida. When you consume olive leaf extract, your body produces enzymes which transform oleuropein into elolenic acid. Elolenic acid strengthens your body's immune system, allowing it to fight off various harmful bacteria, viruses and fungi. According to the renowned olive leaf extract expert, Dr. Morton Walker, olive leaf extract goes far beyond simply slowing the growth of fungi. Instead, it kills fungi at their source and prevents their spread. Unlike many harsh and debilitating anti-candida medical treatments, olive leaf extract is a completely natural and safe substance, which, when used as recommended, will not harm the body's organs or tissues as it kills off the fungi.

How to Use Olive Leaf Extract against Candida:

(**Please Note:** it is always important to first consult with your regular healthcare provider to ensure that any substance you begin taking will not result in any adverse effects, due to interactions with medication you are taking or any existing conditions you may have.)

You will usually find olive leaf extract sold in capsule form. Ensure that the capsules you take are at least 20 percent oleuropein. High oleuropein content will make the capsule much more effective at fighting candida at lower doses

Dosage: The usual dosage of olive leaf extract capsules can range from four to twelve 500 mg capsules of olive leaf extract (with up to 20 percent oleuropein).

Always begin taking supplementation at lower doses and as your tolerance is established, increase dosage slowly, if required.

Candida Die-Off: Because olive leaf extract is such an efficient and potent candida-killer, candida tends to die very quickly once you begin to supplement with this extract. This rapid die-off may be wonderful news for your autoimmune condition and your long term health but it can have some unpleasant short term side effects. These include: Flu-like symptoms such as aches, chills, sweating, nausea, headaches and brain fog. This is only a result of the huge amounts of candida all dying simultaneously and not being eliminated from your body as quickly as they die. The best remedy for this is to rest and drink plenty of pure water in order to allow the dead candida to be flushed from your system naturally. These symptoms typically only last a few days to a week.

Other helpful natural anti-candida remedies include:

(Please Note: Again, consult with your doctor before use to ensure that these supplements are right for you and will not interact negatively with your condition or any medication you're on.)

Garlic: Garlic is a potent fungi and bacteria fighter. As long as you are regularly consuming fresh, raw garlic, candida will have a very difficult time trying to stay alive within your body. I recommend that you avoid taking garlic capsules because raw garlic is much more active and effective.

Oregano Oil: Oregano oil is simply packed with strong, concentrated phenols that can radically reduce levels of candida in the body. Try to use wild oregano oil, as it is more powerful.

Black Seed and Cumin: Both black seed and cumin have similar anti-candida actions and have been used in anti-bacterial, anti-fungal and anti-viral treatments since ancient times. Simply chew a teaspoonful of either black seeds or cumin seeds about half an hour before meals and swallow down with pure water. Make sure your seeds are as fresh as possible and that you take them with ample water. Also be careful not to inhale the seeds accidentally, as they may cause choking. (**Note:** because these two are seeds, do NOT take them during the 7 to 8 weeks of the AIP elimination stage, because all seeds are prohibited during the elimination period. Instead, take them before or after the elimination period.)

Once you weaken and eliminate the candida that has spread systemically throughout your body, you will notice many fantastic changes. Stubborn pounds will begin to naturally disappear, your energy levels will rise and you will see vast improvements in your clarity of though as well as your mood. Even more important than the symptomatic relief that the AIP diet, the use of an anti-candida diet and supplementation with the natural substances above provide, is the knowledge that all of these steps will fight back against the destruction cause d by autoimmune disorders. While many conventional doctors claim that it is impossible to cure autoimmune disorders completely, vast amounts of people who have taken these steps outlined above and use natural therapies such as exercise, vitamin D and relaxation have found that their autoimmune condition improves and does not return.

If you are ready to take your healing out of the hands of doctors and drug companies and instead, take charge of your future, your body and your life, try to follow the elimination diet and anti-candida stages particularly carefully. It is important not to "cheat" while on these treatments because you will only be prolonging your condition and strengthening the severity of autoimmune damage on your tissue.

Now that you've learned how to take some powerful steps to get your AIP and anti-candida diets underway and effectively eliminate the autoimmune threat, join me in the next chapter for a Paleo secret that will have you dropping pounds, gaining health and energy and looking and feeling brand new, with minimal effort!

See you there!

Chapter 15:
The Hunter's Rest: How Sleep Can Give You the Paleolithic Edge You Need

How did you sleep last night? How about the night before that? If you're like millions of Americans, you're surviving on 5 hours or less of fitful, low-quality sleep, fueled only by endless mugs of strong coffee and the knowledge that you HAVE to keep going. You know that a lack of it makes you tired, angry and even sick to your stomach, but just how important is sleep, really? The fact that this chapter is wholly dedicated to the topic of getting ample rest is a testament to sleep's role as a foundation for both mental and physical health as well as longevity.

In earlier chapters, we've gone in-depth about what to eat (and what not to eat) but as mentioned previously, living a truly paleo lifestyle is about far more than just food. It's about making use of the ancient and complete lifestyle solutions that the human body craves and requires. When it comes to accessing the total body and mind health of our hunter-gatherer ancestors, it is absolutely imperative to realize how every factor of our daily lives can affect our wellbeing. These vital factors of our overall health include eating, drinking, exercise and yes, sleep. Sleep is an essential function that allows your body to heal, repair and reset itself, in order to fend off damage and diseases and maintain an optimal level of health, fitness and even happiness. Think about this: The average day is packed with physical, mental and emotional triggers, demands and stressors, exacting a heavy toll on you.

Whether it's dealing with a flood of pollution or other toxins in the environment or battling inflammation spikes in its tissues, your body is perpetually forced to defend itself against the ravages of day to day living. And what allows it to stand up to this constant onslaught? The answer is deep, restful and restorative sleep. Now, I'm not talking about the way that we sleep in these modern times. The brief, disturbed and shallow type of sleep most people manage to receive these days is nothing like the life-giving sleep our ancestors enjoyed in generations past. In fact, over 44 percent of American adults now report experiencing insomnia, finding it difficult or impossible to fall and stay asleep in a meaningful and restorative way. Because of this struggle, we now we see an enormous influx of sleep-loss related conditions and disorders. Everything from rising rates of obesity and uncontrollable appetites to increases in Alzheimer's, Parkinson's and other types of dementia have been linked to a lack of decent quality sleep and are now being seen in younger and younger population groups.

In order to fully understand the risks of poor quality sleep and disrupted sleeping patterns, let's take a look at how sleep impacts the body:

When you achieve deep sleep, you are giving your body many intensely rewarding benefits. Good sleep protects your existing memories and enhances your ability to make and pull up new memories. Why is this important? Well, apart from the purely sentimental value of remembering the good times memory is an essential component in every living thing's survival skills. If you experience negative consequences from a certain action, you learn quickly to avoid those actions and steer a better course. But ONLY if you can remember what you did wrong. Now that may seem simplified but the fact is that this kind of memory-led learning is just as essential in your adult life as it is when you are first taking a step or learning that fire can be harmful. Take, for instance, your interactions at work. How do you learn which strategies are necessary for staying on your boss's good side, closing the deal or managing your relationships with colleagues? By making and keeping memories that allow you to quickly, almost instinctively select and implement the correct behavior almost without thought. In fact, what we so often call instinct would more appropriately be entitled memory-driven strategizing. Without the ability to create, retain and access our memories, we are essentially like newborns, without the skill and tactics we've learned and continue to learn every day in order to survive and thrive. We are no different from our hunter ancestors because although we no longer live in a jungle, we are still faced with a wide variety of challenges, threats and risks in our modern environment, from something as simple as driving or staying healthy enough to do our jobs properly to the rush of chemicals and other toxins in our air, water and food. All of these pose a serious threat to our survival and we all know that when it comes to nature, only the strong survive. This is where the importance of sleep comes in. Sleep allows us to sharpen and maintain the skills that are necessary for us to be able to live and continue to thrive.

Our ancestor, the hunter, needed good quality sleep in order to be able to spring up, awake, aware and ready for any kind of challenge that the wild and unpredictable environment around him could possibly throw his way. In the same way, we also need to be alert, truly rested and ready for anything our modern but no less challenging environment may surprise us with during the course of a day. That's why cultivating proper sleeping habits is nothing less than absolutely vital. It has been said that sleep is the cousin of death but in reality, LACK of sleep is very closely related to failing health, low survival rates and premature death. In fact, sleep deprivation can kill a person much more rapidly than starvation! Let's take a look at this list of sleep-related conditions, disorders and diseases to see just how important sleep really is to every function of our bodies and minds:

Your Brain: Getting the right amount (and quality) of sleep every night is the most meaningful way that you can support your brain's health as well as sharpen and maintain its functions. Put simply, sleep makes your brain work. While your relaxing in the bliss of a good night's sleep, your brain is busily carrying out required repairs, healing damage from the day and preparing you for the day ahead by creating new pathways that help you to access and retain new knowledge. Research has shown that proper sleep greatly improves your ability to learn new information and use this information correctly. From studying for an exam to performing a new task at work, sleep provides you with alertness, the ability to focus and excellent decision making skills and can even enhance your creativity!

On the flip side, data also shows that missing out on deep, high-quality sleep leaves your brain vulnerable to numerous threats. One study even shows that missing sleep consistently can actually SHRINK your brain! Lack of sleep can also change slowdown or even shutdown activity in certain areas of your brain. Just as good sleep directly leads to enhanced decision making, risk assessment ability, problem solving and control of your actions and emotions, sleep deficiency is at the root of poor decision making, inability to properly assess risky situations, lack of problem solving skills and the loss of control and emotional balance. This loss of emotional balance often leads to depressive, angry and even paranoiac symptoms, violent mood swings and aggressiveness, depending on how long the lack of sleep has lasted.

Numerous studies have even shown that a consistent lack of sleep is linked to a rise in suicidal behavior-the exact opposite of the survival-enhancing properties of good sleep! While getting the sleep your body and mind need helps you to function at your highest level, keeping you ultra- sharp, motivated, healthy and positive, losing out on this fountain of mental health can leave you feeling hopeless, goalless and even set off a serious episode of emotional disturbance.

Your Body: A lack of sleep has also been linked to extensive physical deterioration. Because your body uses sleep as an opportunity to repair and heal your heart and blood vessels, going without shut-eye can lead to an onslaught of serious damage and diseases. It's a well-documented fact that continual sleep deficiency can increase your risk of suffering from cardiac disease, kidney disorders, high blood sugar leading to diabetes, high blood pressure, organ failure and stroke. It is very important to take these words to heart. A lack of sleep KILLS, just as surely as smoking several packs of cigarettes a day does. The only difference is that losing out on sleep kills much more quickly than cigarettes do!

Low quality and quantities of sleep are also a major part of the rising obesity epidemic. In fact, studies show that for every individual HOUR of sleep you lose, the chances of your becoming obese shoot up correspondingly! Sleep helps to regulate satiety and hunger signals in the brain but when you miss out on the hours you need, your body remains in constant hunger mode. Even worse, blood sugar levels rise out of proportion, making you hungry for sugary carbohydrates in particular. Add this to the desire to ward off exhaustion by eating and you've got the perfect recipe for a weight gain disaster.

Make no mistake: If you're eating paleo but you're not sleeping well, you're not really paleo at all. To be truly paleo, you need to respect your body's natural desire and need for sleep and you also need to guard your evening routine. Without setting up a solid sleep regime, all of the other healthy life changes you are making with the paleo way of eating will do you very little good. Sleep is as vital as water. Remember that and you'll be far less likely to squander this precious (and FREE!) healing and rejuvenating tool on late night TV or social media. It's precisely because our ancestor, the hunter, did not have these distractions that he could survive the dangerous world around him and remain at the top of the food chain.

If you're ready to make great sleep a priority, then let's take a look at the simple steps below, to help you reap all of the rich rewards of this priceless revitalizer:

1. **Go Outside:** What? Right now? If that's what you're thinking then I have a question for you: Is it light out and is there some sunshine? If you're answer is yes and you haven't gotten at least 15 minutes of sunlight exposure today, then you absolutely need to be out there. The fact is, the way we live now, tied down to

desk jobs under artificial fluorescent lighting makes for a very unhealthy detachment from the natural cycles of dark and light, day and night. Divorced from these shifts, we find ourselves exhausted during the day and unable to sleep in the evening. Our bodies were not designed for this. We should be full of energy and alert during active daylight hunting (or working, driving, living hours) hours and ready to relax into sleep by nightfall. This natural cycle is called the circadian rhythm and it is by this unspoken code that the human body is governed. When we have proper circadian rhythms, we are able to wake up fully rested, feeling that our need for sleep has been thoroughly quenched. We do better throughout the day, using the sharpened thinking and optimized physical health that our sleep has given us and by the time it evening, we effortlessly dial down, unwind and ease into a nourishing night's rest.

Sounds good right? It all starts with getting enough sunlight during daylight hours to let your body know that it is time to be awake and then reducing the amount of light you are exposed to as the day wanes. If you work indoors, you can do this most effectively by getting as much sun as possible during your lunch break (don't forget to use a natural SPF on sensitive areas). If your skin tone is very fair, get no more than 10-15 minutes of direct sun a day and get into the shade when your skin turns slightly pink. If you have olive-toned or darker skin, you can stay in the sun from 30 to 45 minutes, as long as you keep an eye out for reddening skin. If you live in a very sunny climate then you can even fit in some sunlight early in the morning. Remember, our hunter-gatherer ancestors lived and worked in the great outdoors, receiving plenteous amounts of sunlight and fresh air and even today, your body is made to thrive and flourish with similar conditions. Ensure that you get adequate sun and plenty of light during your day and then, around sundown (the exact time will differ depending on your geographical location) start to remove false light from your environment. For example, at home, use dimmers and stay away from bright fluorescent lighting. If your kitchen has fluorescent lighting, switch it off and bring in a lamp with warmer light. If you watch TV or work on the computer during the earlier hours of the evening, make sure you do so with other lights dimmed and perhaps add a few candles, to mimic the calming effect of the cooking fires that our ancestors used to gather around. Your body will instinctively recognize and respond to the flickering flames as a signal to relax and get ready for rest.

2. **Put Away All Artificial Light Sources At Least 1 Hour before You Attempt to Sleep**: This is very important. All of the blinking, beeping devices we surround ourselves with day and night are dangerous culprits behind the dramatic rise in poor sleep quality. Many studies have shown that checking your phone, using your computer or watching TV before sleeping greatly diminishes the quality and quantity of your deep-cycle sleep. This is because the blue light that all of these devices emit has a directly disruptive effect on your body's production of melatonin, the sleep inducing hormone. Inadequate melatonin production is the reason that many cranky, exhausted people these days live off of coffee, fast food and adrenaline and have to struggle to stay awake when that

afternoon slump sets in. If you want all day energy when you *have* to be up and working, make sure that when you *don't* have to be at your computer or awake, you are firm about getting the rest you need. At first, it can be difficult to ignore the nagging feeling that you need to check your email or the desire to catch your usual shows, but after one or two nights of deep, uninterrupted sleep, you won't believe how much health, rejuvenation and revitalization you've been missing out on! Trust me, if the hunter was transported to our modern times for a day, he would be shocked at the way we sacrifice sleep, one of the most essential and powerful survival tools available to us, in order to waste our precious downtime away with silly tasks and recreational activities. Why? Because the hunter knew that lack of sleep meant lack of energy, healing and repair. It translated directly into being so unaware that you could wander into the path of a dangerous animal or being so worn down that you couldn't fend off the many diseases just waiting to take over your system. There was no way that the hunter would risk going out to hunt and gather every day without a full 8 hours or more of real sleep behind him and there should be no way that you venture out to work, live and survive without the same restorative sleep our bodies have always needed.

Keep your cellphone, IPad, reading devices, computers and even that blinking alarm clock out of your bedroom. Our bodies were meant to fall asleep in total blackness so try putting up a pair of blackout drapes for ultimate darkness. Go without watching TV and use those extra hours to lull yourself into deep sleep. Believe me, when you wake up refreshed and energetic the next morning, you'll regret all of the years of non-paleo sleeping patterns you've been damaging your body and mind with!

3. **Keep Cool:** Our ancestors didn't have indoor heating systems or electric blankets. Many of them did not even have the embers of a dying fire to sleep beside. They slept in a relatively unsheltered state because their huts and caves were not sealed and their bodies were forced to reflect the normal drop in temperature that occurs outdoors during the evening hours. Believe it or not, this was a major

bonus for them because the human body can only fall into its deepest level of sleep when its core temperature has dropped sufficiently.

You don't have to freeze to death to get good sleep but you should definitely avoid unnecessarily warm blankets, cranked up thermostats and bulky sleepwear items. With the sealed and sturdy homes we live in these days, you may be wondering if we can ever achieve the natural drop in temperatures required for good sleep. Well, there is a very simple way around this issue that many paleo practitioners and sleep specialists have been using for years.

About an hour before you head to bed, draw yourself a warm bath and enjoy a relaxing soak. When you leave the bath, make sure that your bedroom's temperature has been suitably lowered (cool but not freezing!) and that your bed is not loaded with heavy comforters and blankets. When you go from the warmth of your bath to the relative coolness of your bedroom, your body will naturally mimic the core temperature drop necessary to produce deep, high-quality sleep!

Cultivate these 3 essential habits in order to access the great sleep your body so desperately craves and if you need help starting out, try delicious and sleep-promoting paleo foods such as red meat, eggs, fish, poultry(turkey in particular) and almonds. They are all packed with sleep-inducing tryptophan, a substance that also regulates mood and increases levels of the feel-good hormone serotonin, so enjoy a helping of these foods during dinner and you'll be setting yourself up for the best, most restorative sleep you have ever experienced!

Join me in the next chapter, where we'll look at the powerful ancient secrets of exercise that our ancestors used to give them the upper hand in a wild and challenging world and how you can use these same techniques to survive and thrive. Trust me, you won't want to miss this!

Chapter 16:
How to Move like A Hunter For the Fittest, Slimmest, Healthiest Body Ever!

Have you ever hit the gym faithfully, nearly every day of the week, giving it your maximum effort for an hour or more each time, pounding the treadmill, using the weights and yet, not getting anything like the results you deserve? You are not alone. Millions of people sign up for gym membership, go all out and when they fail to see any real results, end up so discouraged and disappointed that they end up giving up on exercise altogether. What are they doing wrong? They are exercising like machines and not like humans. The theoretical side of exercise has completely take over, making us believe that we should be doing so many reps, so many minutes of running, and so many hours of other cardio workouts that we end up forgetting that our ancestors did not do any of these prescribed workouts and yet, were arguably much healthier, slimmer and fitter than we are today, with a higher proportion of muscle of fat and much better levels of endurance than we could ever muster. Still, when I say move like our ancestor the Hunter, you probably have some doubts. I mean, no one wants to go out stalking potentially deadly wild animals for weight loss and fitness benefits and even if you did, few of us live in environments that offer the opportunity. In any case, that's not necessary. There are plenty of much more achievable and simple ways to get the Paleo results you crave with minimum hassle.

The Principles of Paleo Exercise:

1. Affordability: Paleo exercising is incredibly budget-friendly because it is **absolutely free!** Unlike those pricey gym memberships and fitness plans that require expensive equipment, Paleo exercise is open to all and just as affordable as it would have been during the days that the Hunter roamed the world.

2. Convenience: Most people struggle with modern exercise because, apart from being pricey, it also demands a certain amount of time as well as a particular environment. When it comes to exercising the Paleo way however, none of that is a concern. In fact you can fit in some movement throughout the day, when you have the time and you will be amazed with the results!

3. **Made for Humans, Not Machines:** Unlike those harsh, repetitive and mechanized workouts that so many people suffer through these days, the Paleo way of exercising is based on your body's natural movements and functions. That's why it WORKS for your body, NOT against it.

So now that we understand the basic guiding principles of Paleo exercise, let's get into the nitty-gritty. Don't worry, even if you are an exercise-phobic person, paleo exercise can and will work for you, making it much more natural and instinctive to obtain and maintain amazing results.

1. **Trade Pace for Quantity:** This basically means that our ancient hunter-gatherer ancestors were not doing lots of heart-pumping cardio in the sense of those half-hour, all out sprints that modern trainers push you to do. Instead, they were nomads, long term, low intensity movers who much of the time, kept their heart rate at a nice, steady pace. The best possible rate of movement to mimic the long, loping strides of the average ancient hunter is a rate at which you can still comfortably talk. If you're gasping for breath, you are moving too fast. When

measured, your heart rate should not be hitting levels anywhere above 80 percent. So what works? Moderate to brisk sustained walking is the premium Paleo exercise while jogging or running is not.

2. Moderate Cardio: Take a hike. Seriously, hiking is the perfect imitation of the hunt and stalk movements of our ancient ancestors. Head for an uphill trail and either walk or bike it, keeping your goals focused on duration of movement and not speed. The Hunter may have stalked and hiked for a good portion of his day but he did it all at a very moderate speed.

3. Add Some Weight: Sometimes the Hunter would be forced to carry a heavy animal carcass back to his shelter, through many miles of brush. While I don't advocate carrying dead deer as you hike, you can add a loaded backpack to imitate the difficulty level of the Hunter's hikes.

4. Swim for Duration, Not Speed: If your favorite form of exercise is aquatic, then you're in luck because not only is local pool membership generally cheap-to-free, depending on his geographic setting, the Hunter also spent time in water sources,

cooling off or foraging for food. Just as you do when hiking, remember to focus less on speed and more on getting an evenly-paced workout that still tires you out a bit.

5. **Stand Up:** It really is that simple. Just adding periods of standing instead of sitting throughout your day will help you to access the health and fitness benefits that your on-his-feet ancestor, the Hunter had.

6. **Kick the Chronic Cardio Habit:** Chronically overdoing the cardio can actually break down your body's health and fitness, making you far less likely to lose the amount of weight you desire. Regularly pushing your body too hard, for too long, while doing cardio exercises can result in complete adrenal fatigue and burnout as well as impaired thyroid activity. It can also speed up the aging process through oxidation. If you need proof of this, simply look at the prematurely wizened faces of elite runners and cyclists.

7. Do the Heavy Lifting: Weight machines in gyms simply cannot give you the amazing

muscle tone that our ancestors had. Instead, lift like they did. Instead, utilize objects like dumbbells, large rocks or even your own bodyweight for your true Paleo workout.

Use your bodyweight to do pull ups, pushups, lunges and squats, to recapture the strength that ancient humans cultivated while doing work. Instead of doing hours of weight work and too many reps, space out all lifting exercises over the day to get the best, long, lean muscle mass.

8. Run for It: When our ancestor the Hunter was stalking his prey he would do lots of moderate hiking punctuated by a few bursts of sudden intense activity, as he tried to catch the fast-moving game. Today, we call this High Intensity Interval Training (HIIT). HIIT helps your body to continue to burn calories long after you have stopped exercising, setting up your metabolism for an all-day burn. HIIT should ideally be done for approximately 30 minutes at a time, two times a week in the following way:

High Intensity Interval Training to Get the Optimal Paleo Workout Results:

The Warm Up: Start by warming up with moderate movements for up to 5 minutes.

Burst into Activity: Whether you are running, walking, biking or swimming, burst into the fastest, hardest activity that you can manage for up to 40 seconds.

Return to Moderate Activity: Go back to exercising at a lower, more sustainable speed for 80-90 seconds.

Repeat: Do this at least 7 times and no more than 10 times in a row.

It's Not All Hunting: Our ancient ancestors did more than just hunt prey. They also regularly foraged and gathered foods as well as constructed and repaired shelters. This "work" – style of exercising can be achieved by doing the modern day equivalent- activities such as gardening and common chores like cleaning, sweeping, mopping and vacuuming. These activities should be done to maximize strength with a variety of lunging, squatting and lifting movements. Aim to carry out such activities up to 3 times a week (you probably do so anyway).

Regulate the Amount of Exercise You Get: Let's be clear about this: One of the things that sets Paleo exercising apart from the kind of rigorous but ultimately fruitless modern exercise regimes that so many people fail to thrive on these days, is its focus on quality instead of pointless quantity. Studies have shown that when an individual exercises more than 4 hours a week, they end up harming, instead of helping, their health and fitness. This is because all of those 7 days a week workout regimes cause your body to release huge amounts of the stress hormone cortisol. Cortisol can lead to a slowed -down metabolism and result in weight gin instead of weight loss. Eventually, exercising too much or too intensely ends up burning out the adrenal gland, leading to adrenal fatigue.

This is because human beings were never MEANT to engage in long, protracted physical activity at the highest level of intensity. The Hunter himself could break into high impact activity at any time but would not maintain such intensity over a long period. Any of the marathon runners and gym bunnies of today are actually destroying their physical fitness, straining and damaging their body's tissues and making weight loss impossible to achieve and maintain. Of course, professional athletes and those who are passionate about these high intensity activities may not be willing to give up their long, hard runs and bike rides for good, but simply by reducing the quantity of these actions and giving themselves time to rest and recuperate in between sessions, they can lower their cortisol production and obtain the best possible physical results.

The Paleo Exercise Prescription: For optimal weight loss, fitness and health results, aim to incorporate long, moderately paced or brisk walks along with your Paleo eating plans. Engage in High Intensity Interval Training no more than twice a week and keep your total exercise to no more than 4 hours a week. When used as a part of an all over paleo lifestyle that includes ample sun exposure, proper paleo sleeping techniques and eating an ancestral, intuitive Paleo diet, these ancient ways of moving will totally transform your body, mind and well-being.

Paleo for Life: The Key to Your Strong, Healthy and Happy Future

In closing, I'd like to congratulate you on having comes so far in learning about your health and seeking out the ancient, ancestral ways of eating, living, exercising, sleeping and healing that our ancestors used naturally. If you remain on this path, great health, amazing fitness, long lasting weight loss, increased mental clarity, anti-aging benefits and regulated stabilized moods are all yours to enjoy for a lifetime. Everything in this book is geared towards helping you heal and live your very best life, without expensive pills, treatments or equipment. I'm sure that by now, you've seen just how affordable, easy and effective Paleo living really is.

And one more thing: If you're ever tempted to return to a life of grains, chemicals and bad oils, just remember that it's a jungle out here and only the strong survive! I urge you to use this guide as a reference, to keep yourself on track and remind yourself of all the awesome choices available to you on a revitalizing, rejuvenating Paleo life plan.

And speaking of awesome choices, please enjoy the delicious, naturally nourishing and totally satisfying Paleo recipes that will leave you slim, fit and healthy but won't break the bank, in the mouth-watering Paleo recipe index at the end of this book. These recipes are so flavorful and satiating that you'll never want to go back to non-Paleo eating again!

Now that you are done with living and eating like the prey and instead have become the strong, lean, mean and revitalized hunter that you were always meant to be, allow me to wish you many great years of Paleo success! May you not only survive, but thrive and flourish!

Happy hunting and happy eating!

The Affordable & Delicious Paleo Recipe Index:

These Paleo nutrient-packed delectable recipes are easy to make, easy on your waistline and easy on your budget! What's not to love?

Enjoy in good health!

Paleo Slow Cooker Recipes:

If you're short on time and still want amazing Paleo meals, make the slow cooker your best friend. Slow cooker Paleo meals can help you get a fantastic meal on the table with minimal effort, no waste and all the satisfying Paleo flavors and nutrition your body deserves!

Spicy Slow Cooker Beef Curry:

2 pounds of cubed beef

½ stick of raw milk butter

½ can of pure coconut milk

4 cups of pure chicken broth

4 large yellow onions, chopped up

1 large red bell pepper, chopped up

3 carrots, chopped up

2 chili peppers, diced

3 teaspoons of turmeric

2 teaspoons of freshly minced garlic

3 teaspoons of grated ginger

½ teaspoon of black pepper

½ teaspoon cinnamon

½ teaspoon cloves

Sea salt to season

Steamed cauliflower, reserved

In large pan, brown the beef and onions together in butter

Add beef & onion mix and all other ingredients to slow cooker and allow to cook on low heat for 4 hours

Serve warm over steamed cauliflower

Slow Cooker Sticky Paleo Pork

2 pounds of pork, cubed

1 cup of chopped red onion

2 tablespoons of raw honey

1 teaspoon dried chili flakes

1 red pepper diced

1 teaspoon minced garlic

1/3 cup of beef stock

Sea salt to season

Add all ingredients into the slow cooker and cook for 5 hours. Serve warm.

Legume-Free Paleo Slow Cooker Chili

3 pounds of ground beef or pork

2 cups of diced Portobello mushrooms

½ cup chopped yellow onions

15 oz. of pure roasted tomatoes

10 oz. of pure roasted tomatillos

2 large jalapenos with seeds

1 ½ tablespoons chili powder

2 tablespoons minced garlic

2 teaspoons of cumin

Sea salt and black pepper

Brown up meat and a handful of the onions in skillet

Add all ingredients to slow cooker

Cook for 3 hours

Easy Slow Cooker Chicken Roast

1 whole chicken

3 tablespoons raw butter

1 large green onion, chopped

1 small lemon

2 teaspoons sea salt

1 teaspoon black pepper

Rinse chicken. Pat dry and rub with seasoning and butter.

Slice lemon and place inside chicken's cavity along with chopped green onion. Place in slow cooker and roast on low heat for 4 ½ hours.

Slow Cooker Hearty Paleo Stew

2 cups of water

3 cups of chopped red onions

1 cup of diced spring onions

1 cup of chopped carrots

2 cups of chopped zucchini (or radish, if you can't tolerate zucchini)

1 pound of cubed pork

5 tablespoons pure ghee

3 teaspoons of diced garlic

1 teaspoon cinnamon

3 teaspoons sea salt

Slightly brown pork onions and spring onions, and some garlic with ghee in skillet

Place all ingredients into slow cooker, add seasonings and let cook for at least 5 hours, on low heat. Serve warm in bowls

Sunday Night Chicken Dinner

3 pounds chicken thighs

2 cups of chopped carrots

1/3 cup of chopped yellow onions

5 teaspoons of minced garlic

1 tablespoon of oregano

Sea salt

Pinch of cayenne

½ cup of chicken or vegetable broth

1/3 stick of raw milk butter

Place all ingredients in slow cooker and allow to cook for 3 ½ hours or until tender and fully cooked.

Slow Cooker Pineapple Pepper Pork

1 large pork loin

1/4 cup chicken broth

1/3   cup pineapple slices

2 large green peppers, diced

1 tablespoon minced ginger

2 tablespoons raw honey

2 teaspoons minced garlic

1 teaspoon cayenne pepper

4 tablespoons of coconut oil

Sea salt and black pepper to taste

Make evenly spaced slits all over pork

Rub the pork with coconut oil, garlic ginger, seasoning and honey

Place it with remaining ingredients into slow cooker and allow to cook on low heat for 4-5 hours

Chicken Crock Pot Teriyaki

1 pound chicken cubed

1 ½ tablespoons fresh grated ginger

4 large carrots, sliced

1 large red onion

1/3 cup pure coconut aminos

1 large diced green onion

2 ½ tablespoons of arrowroot flour

Juice of 1 large lemon

1/ 3 cup raw honey

3 tablespoons pure apple cider vinegar

1 tablespoons sesame oil

1 teaspoon cayenne pepper

2 teaspoons minced garlic

Season the raw chicken and place with all ingredients into the slow cooker. Allow to cook for 5 hours, on low heat.

Crock Pot Chicken Chili

1 ½ pounds of chicken

2 large tomatoes

2 large bell peppers

4 tablespoons beef tallow

2 diced yellow onions;

½ of a diced red onion

1 cups pure roasted tomatoes

2 teaspoons minced garlic

2 cups of water

1 teaspoon cilantro

2 ½ teaspoons ground cumin;

3 teaspoons cayenne pepper

Sea salt to season

Black pepper to season

Brown chicken in skillet with onions, beef tallow, bell peppers and seasoning Place this mixture and all other ingredients in the slow cooker and cook on low heat for 4 to 5 hours

Brisket Crock Pot Meal

2 pounds of brisket

1 large yellow onion

2 large carrots

1 ½ cup chicken stock

1 bunch of parsley

2 teaspoons minced garlic

1 teaspoon cinnamon

Sea salt and black pepper to season

Chop carrots, onion, parsley and coarsely and put them in slow cooker .Add stock and put the brisket in slow cooker. Cook for 7 hours on low heat. Serve with all of the juices from the cooker.

Baked Herb-Crusted White Fish

4 large white fish fillets

2 tablespoons olive or coconut oil

2 teaspoons thyme

1 teaspoon dill

1 large lemon sliced

Sea salt to season

Rub fish fillets with olive oil and sprinkle with herb and sea salt

Place lemon slices on fish

Line a baking tray with parchment paper and place fish on it. Bake for approximately 20 minutes.

Steak Dinner "Splurge "

1 pound of a less pricey, fattier cut of beef

1/3 stick of raw milk butter

4 cloves of diced garlic

Sea salt and fresh ground pepper

Steamed and well mashed cauliflower

Slice beef into steaks and place on sizzling grill, without removing fat

Season each side as the other cooks

Remove from grill rare to medium rare and place on top of cauliflower mash

Melt butter and garlic together and spoon over steak before serving

Ground Beef Avocado Cups

4 large ripe avocadoes

1 ½ half ground beef

1 small red onion

2 teaspoons minced garlic

2 tablespoons beef tallow

1 small red pepper, finely diced

1 large lime

Sea salt and cilantro to season

Combine beef, onion, garlic and red pepper and some salt and cilantro and brown in beef tallow in skillet

Slice avocadoes length wise and spoon ground beef mixture into them

Season and squeeze lime juice over them.

Warm Bacon Avocado and Spinach Salad Bowl

2 rashers of non-nitrate bacon

1 large ripe avocado, peeled and cubed

2 bunches of spinach leaves, washed

1 small yellow onion, finely chopped

Dressing:

2 tablespoons raw milk butter

1 teaspoon minced garlic

1 teaspoon of cayenne pepper

Juice of half lemon

Lightly brown the bacon in a skillet and allow bacon to cool slightly before chopping coarsely

In a bowl combine spinach leaves avocado, onion and chopped bacon

In a saucepan melt butter slightly and add garlic cayenne, sea salt

Remove from heat and add lemon juice

Whisk thoroughly and ladle over salad

Paleo Egg Dishes: Eggs make for fantastic Paleo protein and nutrition sources that are as affordable as they are delicious. Check out these easy, tasty and versatile egg dishes that are so irresistible, you'll be whipping them up for breakfast, lunch or dinner!

No-Crust Egg and Mushroom Mini-Quiches

5 oz. of a pure crumbly white cheese

½ cup whole fat raw milk

14 oz. of washed, diced Portobello mushrooms

1 tablespoon fresh dill

3 tablespoons olive oil

1 teaspoon sea salt

1 teaspoon black pepper

1 small scallion, chopped

7 whole eggs

Pre-heat your oven to 375 F and oil your muffin tins with portion of olive oil

Mix cheese, milk, eggs, ad seasoning until creamy and smooth

Sautee mushrooms, dill and scallions in skillet with olive oil

Spoon this mix into muffin tins

Pour egg, cheese, milk mix on top of mushroom mic

Bake quiches for no more than 30 minutes and serve soft and hot

Budget Tip: Store leftover quiches in foil in the fridge for up to a week and reheat in your toaster oven for a quick, satisfying and budget-friendly meal!

Spinach Egg Frittata

6 large eggs, whisked

1 bunch of spinach, washed

1 small scallion

1 tablespoon of olive or coconut oil

3 large pats of raw milk butter

Sea salt and black pepper

In small sauce pan, lightly sauté spinach and scallion in oil

In another pan, melt butter and pour in eggs, seasoning and spinach. Remove from stove top immediately and finish cooking in pre-heated oven or toaster oven until not runny.

Spanish Bacon Scramble

1 rasher non-nitrate bacon

6 large eggs, whisked

1 red onion, chopped

2 cloves garlic, minced

1 teaspoon cumin

¼ of stick of raw milk butter

1 bell pepper, chopped

1 red pepper, finely diced

Sea salt and black pepper

In sauce pan, brown bacon and add bell pepper, red pepper, cumin and garlic

In another pan, melt butter and add whisked eggs and seasoning before adding bacon mix and combining.

Serve warm.

Stewed Paleo Collard Greens

3 bunches of collard greens, washed

½ cup of beef broth

1 cup water

3 tablespoons of beef tallow

1 yellow onion, coarsely chopped

Sea salt and chili pepper to season

In a large pot, stew the collard greens in water and broth until soft. Add beef tallow, onion, sea salt and chili and cover with lid, allowing greens to cook down further. Use as a side to any Paleo main dish.

Full Fat Meatballs and Zucchini Noodles

4 large zucchinis (if tolerated), washed and sliced into noodles

½ pound of fatty ground beef or pork

1 small diced onion

3 cloves diced garlic

4 tablespoons olive or coconut oil

1 bunch roughly chopped parsley

2 large sweet tomatoes

2 teaspoons oregano

4 tablespoons of full fat pure crumbly cheese

Sea salt and freshly ground black pepper

Form ground beef or pork, seasoning and diced onions into meatballs. In large deep pan, heat oil and brown meatballs

Lower heat and add diced sweet tomatoes, garlic, and oregano

Pile zucchini noodles into pan and mix over low heat, season and serve with cheese crumbled over top

Paleo Beverages and Desserts: They may not be the sickly sweet sodas and snacks that the modern day diet is so full of but these paleo drink and dessert options will tantalize your taste buds and satiate all your cravings, while keeping you slim, trim, lean and full of vibrancy!

Beverages:

Citrus Medley

1 small lime

Half of a ripe orange

Half of a lime

1 pitcher of pure water

1 empty pitcher

Wash and slice lemon, lime and orange into thin discs and place them in the freezer. Remove when frozen and fill the empty pitcher. Pour water over the frozen slices and let flavors steep

Pour into glasses and serve

Fresh Cucumber Water

1 large cucumber

1 pitcher of water

Empty pitcher

Wash and slice cucumber into discs and place in empty pitcher

Pour fresh water over them and place in fridge to chill before serving

Fresh Strawberry Water

½ cup of ripe sweet strawberries

1 pitcher of water

1 empty pitcher

1 dash of sea salt

Combine all ingredients in pitcher and stir

Chill to serve

Tart Berry Water Fizz

1/3 cup of raspberries, frozen

1.3 cup of strawberries, frozen

1/3 cup of ripe blueberries or blackberries, frozen

2 liters of fizzy, pure mineral water

Pour all berries into a large pitcher

Pour the fizzy water over the berries

Allow mixture to blend and serve cool

Strawberry Ginger Spinach Smoothie

½ cup of sweet strawberries (fresh or frozen berries are equally good)

1 handful of spinach leaves

1 teaspoon of freshly grated ginger

Juice of ½ a lime

1cup coconut milk (Or if you can tolerate dairy, full-fat, non-pasteurized, grass-fed dairy, cream or yogurt)

Blitz all ingredients together in a blender and serve over ice cubes in tall chilled glasses

Paleo Desserts That Are Nutritious, Nourishing and Ultra-Healthy!

Don't believe it? Just try out these recipes below and give yourself a well-earned treat for all your hard hunting!

Homemade Paleo Coconut Yogurt (This dessert is also approved on the AIP)

2 quarts of pure sugarless coconut milk

1/3 teaspoon of pure yogurt starter

Handful of ripe raspberries or strawberries, washed and sliced lengthwise

Place coconut milk in the stove and gently heat to no more than 107 F

Mix in 1/3 teaspoon of pure yogurt starter

Pour into blender and blend

Pour blended coconut milk and yogurt starter into yogurt maker

Allow mixture to ferment for 14 hours

Cool in the fridge and add berries to serve

Very Berry Paleo Freeze

1 cup of pure coconut milk

2 pints of chilled berries of your choice

2 teaspoons of pure real vanilla (not extract or essence)

2 sprigs of fresh mint

Pour all ingredients into the blender and pulse together

Freeze mixture in freezer until slushy

Garnish with mint and Serve immediately

Fresh and Fatty Avocado Smoothie

2 large ripe, peeled avocadoes

½ cup pure unsweetened coconut milk (fermented, if you wish)

Handful of ice cubes

2 sweet apples, cored and chopped

Juice of ½ a lemon

Blitz all ingredients together in blender until creamy/slushy

Serve in chilled glasses

THE END